Kathlene —
May your journey
be a great joy)
Blessings
[signature]

Awaken
Your Power
to Heal

by Ned Wolf

THE THERAPEUTAE

PRESS

AWAKEN YOUR POWER TO HEAL

by Ned Wolf

Published in the United States by:

The Therapeutae Press
P.O. Box 1557
Bothell, WA 98041-1557
(425) 487-4346

ISBN: 0-9675575-0-X

Cover design: Jerry Downs
Editorial consultant: Tam Mossman

10 9 8 7 6 5 4 3

THE THERAPEUTAE

PRESS

CONTENTS

HEALING YOUR WORLD

What Can We Accomplish Together?

This book is a wonderful collaboration with the many clients and students I have the honor to serve. So many times their own healing experiences opened deep, new insights into my own growing. These pages represent many of the gifts of our working together.

I've changed clients' identities, yet very probably you'll recognize your own stories among those I've presented here.

To all those whose lives have contributed to this work, I thank you. AWAKEN YOUR POWER TO HEAL is dedicated to all family, friends and clients woven into the folds of these pages. I thank each of you, with deep, heartfelt gratitude.

This book presents many tools, useful in claiming your birthright to heal. I've sought to clarify the incredible power to create available within each of us, and illustrate many of the more obvious ways we resist that power. My intention is that you discover richer, more effective uses of your own creative energies.

Using these ideas fully will transform your relationship with energy and thus, your relationship with yourself and the world around you.

Few of us today believe in a flat world, or are employed in the manufacture of buggy whips. Discrimination is not socially acceptable. History is the story of the evolution of consciousness. Yes, we would all wish our growth to occur more rapidly, more gently. Yet, as we've grown past limitations, our struggles become a part of humankind's unique heritage.

Sometimes I like to poke fun at our collective resistance to our own growth. I know I've seen myself look downright silly as I argue for my own blind spots. We have yet to overcome our control games around pain and conflict. Our dependence on these blind spots has undermined our relationships with our own physical health, with those we love and with those we share the planet.

Woven through my stories, clients' histories and the resultant fabric of ideas are a number of exercises I have found useful in the exploration of growth and healing. Please consider all these exercises as experimental. Focus on them, work with them, and see which ones produce results. Those that do, make them your own. Those that don't, throw out and continue exploring.

This way, you allow your own experience to teach you, and you expand your own authority for your own choices. True economy— for you have just saved yourself the trouble of needing to create yet another outside authority.

Take this book slowly. Give it time to replace other, more familiar hypnotizers in your life. After you've read a chapter (or even a segment), go out and shake up your personal universe.

It's easy— you can start by changing your patterns of living. Buy a journal for the exercises coming up. Make your television a planter box! Walk in nature. Share a fond memory with a neighbor you don't know well. As you use this book, be willing for the experience to transform your life. If you're not willing to make that kind of commitment right now in your life, fine—simply pass this book along to someone else. And bless yourself.

As you explore these ideas, let them challenge you. Examine your own self-imposed limitations, and find out what they're costing you. Let them teach you more about healing. Tear out the pages, write in the margins. Drop this book on the floor, and then read the pages where it falls open. Photocopy exercises and send them as letters to your family.

I encourage you to pretend these pages are prayers. Read them out loud, or sing them. Write me with your questions;

Or simply try to convince me that you aren't a magnificent, unique, unlimited expression of God.

Blessssings,
Ned Wolf

CHAPTER ONE
A New Client

Rounding the corner into the entry of my offices in Seattle, I encountered a surprise. The stranger in front of me was an attractive, successful looking woman, but as she walked through the sunlit foyer, she carried herself with hesitancy, perhaps even fear.

Sometimes clients remind me of dogs who have been disciplined too harshly — slouching along with their tails between their legs. Since all of my clients are referred by other people I've worked with, I'm reasonably certain that whoever shows up in my office is going to have problems. Still, I'm always surprised and a bit concerned when people carry themselves with such reticence— especially when they have as much going for them as this woman apparently did.

"Welcome." I smiled and held out my hand.

She tentatively allowed me to shake hers. "Hi," she said softly, "I'm Anne." Her tone of voice told me she was frightened, and her gaze was begging me to be gentle. From my 14 years as a counselor, I knew that Anne must be facing some pretty powerful demons to find herself in such a state.

"Would you like a cup of tea?" This is my standard protocol to help put new clients at ease. "Let's go into the back office, where we can talk."

Anne waited as I poured the tea, then followed me down the hall. Like most new clients who step into my inner office, she lit up when she saw the archway that looks out the window into the courtyard. She stopped in front of the large pane of glass, watching the morning's flock of sparrows thronging the feeder. "A squirrel!" she exclaimed. The furry acrobat had just leaped from the plum tree across the courtyard to the fence, carrying away one of the peanuts I left for him that morning.

After we sat down, I talked a bit about my feeding the animals in the courtyard. Anne's shoulders started to relax. Then I explained to her how I operate: "I'm going to treat you as though you're a powerful, unlimited being," I began. "You may not always agree with me, but I'm going to take the point of view that you had a hand in creating all the trouble, pain, and conflict in your life. And, since you created it, I also assume that you're entirely capable of healing any imbalance. In fact, I believe it'll take you less energy to restore balance than it took to create the original imbalance in the first place."

She nodded.

"I'm not here to fix you or heal you or make you feel better," I went on. "Why would I do that, when you already have the power to do so? And I certainly don't want to take the joy of discovering that power away from you."

Anne nodded, listening. She relaxed her shoulders a bit more and sat back in the chair.

"And if you don't experience results by working with me, then it's your job to fire me. We'll find someone else with whom you can work who will be more effective."

At that, she even chuckled.

"Anne, I want *you* to heal whatever's troubling you. My commitment is to bring all my knowledge, talents and abilities to serve that purpose. And I ask a commitment of you: that you be willing to wade into whatever swamp we encounter. Face whateve alligators you've put there. Also, I ask that you don't leave this healing process while you're in the middle of the swamp!"

Anne hesitated, and turned her attention inward. She was considering the pain she was carrying, asking herself, *Can I really face this?* For a moment, she debated silently, her eyes never leaving mine. Then she said simply, "Okay." I could see that Anne had committed to her own healing!

"Great," I exclaimed. "What would you like to say about what's troubling you?"

She began by telling me about Jack, her truck-driving husband, who was becoming more and more critical in their relationship. "He seems to complain a lot about all the time I spend grooming our pets and riding horses," she explained. "He often gets upset that I can't spend more time with him after work. Jack doesn't seem to understand that being a law office administrator, and the mother of a four-year-old, doesn't leave me lots of time to help him remodel our home."

As I expressed encouragement, Anne went on to voice her concerns for their son, Luke, who was beginning to withdraw from his father. Jack seemed to become more irritable whenever Luke didn't meet his father's expectations.

Anne's scenario resembled many others I'd heard about: Her high-pressure job where she often felt the need to complete others' tasks; a semi-absent husband; a home on Whidbey Island that necessitated three-hours of commuting every day, including dropping her son off at a day care center near her office in Seattle. Whatever the source of Anne's pain, I could tell that the stress of trying to accommodate her lifestyle wasn't helping much.

But as we talked, I could see that she was becoming fearful. "Maybe," I said, "we can interrupt our conversation and initiate a process whereby you can explore the sensations you're feeling."

Anne agreed. Asking her to close her eyes, I led her through an exercise of breathing and focusing on exactly where she felt the fear in her body. As she described the experience, I asked, "Would you be willing to love yourself in the midst of the fear?"

Suddenly, she broke down crying. Anne revealed that she had great apprehension about even talking about her marital problems—for fear she would lose her son!

"Jack says I need to quit my job and find work on the island," she sobbed, "or else he'll divorce me and take custody of Luke, and I won't be able to see him."

In Washington State, the courts generally award residential rights to a young child's mother. Given Anne's care and concern for Luke, it just didn't add up that Jack could become his custodial parent. Tangled somewhere within Anne's anxiety, there had to be some failed expectation or guilt, leading her to question her worth as a mother.

"Anne," I asked quietly, "do you believe that somehow you're being a bad mom?"

Her face contorted in anger. "Jack's always telling me that," she exclaimed. I gave her a chance to vent, and she continued for some time, releasing quite a lot of pent up frustration and resentment about the pejorative names Jack had called her, the accusations he made, and his threats to take Luke away.

Gently, I inquired whether Anne had experienced any physical abuse. No, Jack had never committed violence, nor even threatened it! Reassured, I decided to probe deeper.

In my own relationship with anger, and with hundreds of clients, I've learned that deeply held resentments are signals that, in some way, we haven't been expressing our true wants and desires. In intimate relationships, often we put our own needs on the back burner, trying to avoid conflict and anger with our partner. The resultant resentments we often blame on our partner.

Anger is a sign that something vital is missing. Over the years, in sessions with clients, I've regularly used the presence of anger as an effective healing tool. Of all the painful feelings we experience, anger is among the easiest to unlock. We can use it to explore why we blame others for our troubles, rather than considering that same pain as an internal messenger that cannot only help heal us, but also help us create what we really want out of life.

I had an inkling that within their sexual relationship, Anne might be not speaking up for herself. "Anne," I asked quietly, "would you please tell me about the physically intimate part of your marriage?"

"Well . . ." she hesitated. "We make love two or three times a week."

"Okay . . . and who initiates the contact?"

"Jack."

"Always?"

"Yes."

"And," I asked softly, "how do you feel about making love to Jack?"

"I don't want to," she said, matter-of-factly.

"Does Jack know this?"

"No." Here, we'd uncovered at least one source of Anne's pain. For the rest of the session, we talked about ways she could begin to communicate to her husband how she truly felt. I suggested that she ask him to understand that she wanted to discover how she could grow, and encourage him to be patient. I suggested that she tell him, "Jack, I'll probably change, and our relationship needs to change and grow as well." I suggested she start speaking up for herself more and tell Jack that she didn't always enjoy their lovemaking—but I suggested that she hold this conversation with him outdoors, not in their bedroom.

Finally, I suggested she bring Jack in for a joint session. After reviewing the communications exercises I'd suggested for homework, we scheduled her next appointment.

A week later, Anne returned, looking slightly more energetic. As we sat down, I asked, "How did the communication exercises go?" She admitted that she'd tried only once, and gave up after Jack became even more judgmental and made fun of her decision to begin counseling.

Faced with the threat of losing her child, a mother will move heaven and earth to prevent it. Since Anne had given up on her homework after only one try, I sensed there was more to discover about of the source of her pain.

During this session, she revealed her first love: "I've always wanted to work with animals. I've retained this administrator's job because I need the money to maintain our family's real estate holdings and to cover expenses whenever Jack goes through sparse times as a trucker." The more Anne talked, the more obvious it became that she felt trapped, and blamed Jack as the reason.

"Anne," I said, "do you know the single most powerful way to block healing?" I could see I had her attention.

"No," she replied.

"Blame. Whenever we hold someone else as the cause of our pain, we get stuck in the pain. As long as we believe someone else must change before we can get back in balance, we can't heal pain. Blame blocks healing!"

"So," asked Anne, "how does that relate to me? After all, it's Jack who accuses me—and then blames me for his anger."

"Well, Anne," I said as gently as I could. "You will recall, I consider you a powerful being. So let's explore what other emotions you might be having in your relationship with Jack. How are you feeling now?"

"I'm getting angry," she said tersely.

"Would you be willing to do that healing exercise we began last week?"

"Okay," she said.

Once again, we began with Anne closing her eyes and taking deep, connected breaths, with no pauses between each successive inhale and exhale.

"While you're breathing, tell me where in your body the sensation of anger seems to be most obvious." We walked through the physical experiences of her anger. "Now . . . Anne? Ask the anger if it has a message for you."

She paused for a moment, listening internally. "I'm feeling ashamed," she said in a very small voice. Once again, I could see tears starting to flow.

"Do you use anger to hide your shame from yourself? Does that fit?"

"Yes!"

"Anne, do you know what you're ashamed of?"

"My drinking," she meekly replied.

"Thank you, Anne. You can open your eyes now." I knew she'd just revealed a wellspring of shame that she was using, very probably subconsciously, to justify Jack's abusive behavior.

For the rest of the session, we talked about her history of alcohol abuse, and her many failed attempts to be free of her addiction. As she spoke, Anne realized that her relationship with alcohol lay behind the self-destructive, too-accommodating behaviors in her sexual relationship with Jack. To compensate for her own self-judgments as an unworthy drunk, she'd been trying to placate him with physical intimacy.

Once again, we worked the healing/breathing process on Anne's shameful feelings. She discovered that she'd formed destructive judgments around her drinking, reflecting her childhood attitudes about both of her parents' consumption of alcohol.

I suggested to her that addiction was just as valid as any other lesson that the rest of us are being taught—one of the most painful lessons, perhaps, but valid nonetheless: "Maybe no lesson on earth can be any bigger than the person who's learning it. Can you take on the job of loving and validating yourself as you work your way through this lesson?"

Anne was incredulous. Like most clients, she couldn't believe that the fastest way to learn was by accepting and loving herself. Like most of us, she'd been taught to punish herself in order to make any progress. Now, though, she was beginning to see that her judgments and self-condemnation only prolonged the problems.

In subsequent sessions, Anne and I talked about the real issue behind addictions and dependencies—which, I've learned, are simply the denial of a person's own unique expressions, talents and contributions. The more we explored this idea, the more she came to see how much she'd discounted her deep desire to care for animals.

"I just don't see how I can make enough money doing what I love," she complained at one point.

"Would you be willing to experiment, and give it a try for six months?" I knew full well what the outcome would be. "Maybe accepting yourself and doing what you love is worth whatever income reduction you'll experience. Is there any greater legacy you'd rather leave your son?"

By this time, I'd had the chance to work with Jack for several sessions, helping him learn to heal the anger he carried about his wife's drinking. He was very happy to see her progress, gradually at first, with a few relapses thrown in. Yet over time, he found ways to deal with his own pain without verbally attacking his family.

Last I heard, Anne was working at home and, during her spare time, was helping Jack build a barn to accommodate the horses they were boarding. She and Jack had learned that their pain was not their enemy. They found ways to talk about it, without blaming each other as its source. They let themselves accept it, learning to hear whatever unexpected message it had to deliver. Once they came to trust that they each had the birthright of self-healing, they dropped their habit of blame for good and found they could focus on what each of them want out of their relationship and their lives.

Once in a while, they visit my office to work out a conflict. They're still learning how to love themselves—even in the middle of their mistakes. But they've put their family back on the road to growth, nurturing each other and a healthy child.

Over my years of counseling, I've seen clients use this same technique—accepting their pain—to heal a lifetime's worth of internal emotional baggage. As Anne and Jack learned, pain is simply a messenger telling us of a distortion in our perspective.

Too often, we've been taught to believe that problems and imbalances are beyond our ability to handle. It surprises people to hear that they can have a relationship with their pain and communicate with it effectively, but time and time again, they prove that they can.

My job is not to heal them, but to assist them in healing themselves. I want them to leave my office sessions with a greater awareness of their own authority as the prime healer in their lives, rather than try to hand that authority to me. Working through over a thousand client sessions each year, I continually reinforce the discovery that we each hold the keys to our own healing—and that we're meant to access healing in very simple and effective ways.

CHAPTER TWO

Thirty Years of Learning

My move to the Pacific Northwest had been propitious. Not only was I enjoying the beauty of nature—the jagged outline of the Cascade Mountains, the mild winters and spring flowers that erupted in early February, the mist-shrouded ferries plying Puget Sound. Even better, my work was recognized and appreciated.

At 36, I was a hard-working communications director for one of Seattle's largest advertising agencies. Management loved me because I put in long hours and related well to their corporate and financial clients.

One evening, about a dozen people from the agency attended an awards dinner atop the Columbia Tower, where I received their first regional award for a statewide editorial board program I'd written for a banking client. After the presentation my friend Rick, who worked for a competing agency, emerged from the crowd.

"Well, Ned, now that you've won this award, what are you going to do with the rest of your career?"

"If I have to do this for the rest of my life," I responded instantly, "I'm going out to shoot myself!" Listening to my own words, I was shocked to realize that I needed to do more with my life.

I had grown up in rural Colorado, the second oldest in a Catholic family of eight children. My brother is eight years younger, and I was mostly uncomfortable with my six sisters. To avoid the teasing and conflict that often defined our relationships, I frequently isolated myself. Many early mornings, I would ride my bike four miles into town to serve as an altar boy at the day's first Mass. Later, I'd hike the hills alone with our family's hunting dogs. I did relish being outdoors, investigating a wide variety of plant and animal life and enjoying lots of physical activity.

Believing that I had little to contribute, I often found myself at loose ends. The right thing to do, I felt, was to follow my mother's plans for me: attend Annapolis and become a naval officer, as my grandfather had.

My Dad worked as an executive in a marketing corporation. Yet on evenings and weekends, he took the time to teach me to hunt and fish and do chores around the house and barn. He was an active father during the years I spent in Scouting. He and I shared a love for nature and enjoyed camping together. He encouraged several of my sisters and me to play music, a talent I still enjoy, memorizing jazz pieces and playing them on a soprano sax.

One summer morning, I watched my father walk to his car to drive to work. Seeing how he was carrying himself, I realized how unhappy he was about the daily grind. He wasn't going out into the world with the same zest and enthusiasm I saw whenever we took the dogs out hunting, or when we all played music together. Shocked at this realization, I felt very disappointed in him. How could my own father not make a living by doing something he enjoyed?

From that moment, I began kicking apart the pedestal I'd set up for my Dad. Even so, I found this memory tremendously helpful in planning my own future: I was determined to make my career reflect my strongest values—and my deepest loves.

Despite my good grades at the University of Colorado, I was troubled to find that few of my courses captured my imagination.

Once again, I had to cope with a deep desire to isolate myself from other people. It seemed that whenever I tried to deal with my unexplained feelings of guilt and unlovability, I merely created more pain for myself.

The year was 1968. Martin Luther King, Jr., and Robert F. Kennedy had been assassinated. In a world that made no sense, what did I have to contribute? Despairing, I dropped out of college and moved to Glenwood Springs, a fairly remote town high in the Rocky Mountains, almost due west of Denver. I shunned alcohol, but my regular marijuana habit helped distract me from my self-imposed isolation.

While living in the mountains, I found an old Yashica range finder camera and with it, delighted in capturing nature on film. As a boy I'd had little interest in photography, even though it was one of my mother's favorite hobbies. Whenever she pointed her camera at me, I wanted to hide. Now, surprisingly, I enjoyed being on the other side of the lens.

Studying photography at a junior college in Glenwood, I found I'd inherited my mother's powerful sense of composition. That, combined with sufficient technical skill, enabled me to support myself as a freelance photographer for seven years.

When the est training was offered in nearby Aspen, I decided to try it. I found the experience grueling and unreasonable, yet also discovered there were parts of myself that went beyond my beliefs. I found that I didn't have to be ruled by my feeling unlovable—that was a feeling, not a headline statement about myself. And I was excited at the notion that my judgments for my failings had never helped me progress beyond those mistakes. That taught me that I could face my own pain and accept myself just as I was, rather than trying to twist myself into someone whom other people might approve. Best of all, I rediscovered my enthusiasm for living.

Over the next ten years, I continued assisting with est. Ultimately, I was trained to lead seminars, which I did—though not very successfully—in Aspen and New York City. Meanwhile, I enjoyed the freedom of working as a professional photographer, yet was driven to be even more creative.

I began offering editorial and copywriting services to clients, freelancing for local and regional publications in Colorado, covering everything from electric automobiles to the annual stock show. I had exhibitions of my nature photography. I shot portraits for the covers of Denver's business magazines. I wrote marketing copy for small companies—anything to help pay the bills and build my portfolio.

Seven years later, upon arriving in New York, I visited every publication in town looking for work. Finally, after three months of pounding the pavement, I parlayed my freelance reporter's experience into a job as an associate editor for a financial newsletter—which featured high stress, low pay and management with a definite attitude. Despite my complaining about what I considered grueling conditions and my unhappiness with the East Coast life style, the tight deadlines certainly helped me learn to write.

After three years of trying to get out of New York, I succeeded in landing the communications director's job in Seattle. Yet now, after the years of being highly regarded and winning the regional award, I found that I was about to commit the same soul-deadening mistake my father had made. Despairing that my life would never be truly rewarding, I kept thinking back to my reply to Rick at the awards presentation: *If I have to do this for the rest of my life, I'm going to shoot myself!*

I wasn't suicidal, but it would kill me, I knew, if I had to continue writing press releases and communications programs. In all of the jobs I'd held, I'd most appreciated my relationships with the people around me. My life needed to revolve around supporting individuals, not promoting businesses and corporations. I wanted (needed!) to use my heart as well as my mind. My passion lay in making people bigger and the world smaller.

To fulfill that goal, I had to find some way out of the rat race.

Then I met George, a counselor and teacher who had been passionately studying the Essenes, an ancient Jewish sect renowned for their library of ancient Dead Sea scrolls. I was searching for a deeper spiritual life, and George, a graying and grizzled therapist who had been through two wars and at least as many heavy addictions, spoke to me of the Essene way of reclaiming the spirit.

For the next three years, I absorbed many Essene teachings. I learned natural healing, counseling, and various ways to bring my own spiritual connection into my work. (In the Essene tradition, the physical domain was considered to be integral to the spiritual, and I found myself linking my deep love of nature with an inner dimension of wisdom and love.) After studying many healing methods, I gravitated toward spiritual counseling, energy healing and Reiki.

Many ancient cultures, including the Essenes, had healing traditions involving the breath. They considered the air to be a sacred messenger of the physical universe, often sending us subtle messages needed for our own healing and growth. As in yoga, meditation and the martial arts, practitioners used breath to release stress and center themselves. Today, of course, we know of the tremendous role that breathing plays in releasing toxins from the body—but the ancients knew that deep breathing helps release toxins from the mind.

In the course of my studies I was trained as a Rebirther, a breathing therapy developed by Leonard Orr in the sixties. Rebirthing is a powerful tool in resolving deeply held emotional conflicts. During one training session, I came face to face with some deep-seated guilt in my relationship with my mother. I had been feeling badly about rejecting my alternate appointment to Annapolis and disappointing my Mom's hopes for my naval career. Now, though, as I explored that pain, the breathing exercises led me to a memory of being in my mother's womb, just before birth. Many people would argue that infants are barely conscious, yet the countless rebirthings I've experienced provide compelling evidence that we're sentient beings, even in the womb.

Re-experiencing my birth, I discovered deep feelings of guilt, stemming from the assumption that my mother's pain in labor was all my fault. While allowing myself to breathe and accept that emotion, I realized that by getting entangled in guilt, I had missed experiencing all the love available to me when I was born. As I became conscious of that love, the guilt melted away. I was aware of a level of joy that I'd never known before. Today, as a result of this experience, I can support clients in learning to heal their pain, when they explore their own characteristic patterns of guilt and self-blame.

I set out on my own, as a counselor ordained in the Essene Healing Ministries, a non-denominational organization inspired by Essene teachings. But as the months wore on, I saw only four or five clients weekly. I began to despair that I wasn't effective in supporting others in solving their problems. Finally I promised myself that if I didn't have my practice up and running within three months, I'd go out and get a "real" job. (I could always go back to my old position at the ad agency, albeit with my tail between my legs.)

As I sought ways to let people know about my work, I had to face my reluctance to return to giving seminars. Although I'd received the world's best training, I didn't like leading the est seminars that Werner Erhart had put together. They had no connection with spirituality and too much inducement to enroll others. Knowing I had some unresolved pain about leading groups, I took the risk of offering a four-week workshop on self-love. To my surprise, it was well-attended and well-received. Participants wanted counseling and healing, and soon became clients. Before I knew it, I was leading three support groups—and learning from each new client who entered my door.

One evening, I heard a radio ad for conflict mediation training. Within the year, I was certified as a mediator. The Dispute Resolution Center often scheduled me to mediate on a volunteer basis, since my schedule was flexible, and I was willing to confront the heavy emotional climate of families in trouble. I could best support people in pain, I found, by suggesting that they accept the validity of their experiences.

In one particularly acrimonious divorce case, the wife spent a considerable part of her time berating her very angry husband. "I understand that you're upset and hurting," I finally interjected, "but do you realize you can express your pain without attacking your spouse?"

The two looked at each other, shocked and ultimately very relieved. Without further battle, they went on to resolve the impediments to parenting their kids. It was a great joy to watch people naturally moving into resolution and healing.

To help my clients and workshop participants, I continued to follow my curiosity and discovered even more healing methods—herbs, homeopathics and radionics, which I still employ in my current practice today. I teach students about natural healing and spiritual counseling, even as I explore effective new directions for healing myself. (But I don't want you to think my stories are all that important. You've got plenty of significant stories of your own!)

PART ONE

Starting at the Top

Accepting the Power of *Your* Mind,
Your Choice to Focus,
and *Your* Power to Heal

CHAPTER THREE

Thought and Focus — Their Unlimited Power

A s George was teaching, he would often say, "As we think, so do we feel, so do we react or respond—so do we behave." What George meant, I've come to learn, is that when we want to discover the cause of some unwanted feeling or behavior, we first must discover—and change—the thinking that's producing that condition.

Steve, a therapist, was taking a doctor's prescription for anti-depressants. He came to me after one of my clients told him that I had a no-nonsense approach and quickly got to the core of a problem. Steve told me about his failing practice, a bad business investment that was draining his finances, and a growing problem with alcohol. For about forty-five minutes, I just let him talk, listening to his words and tone of voice, noticing how he presented himself. Aside from a few brief glances, he couldn't look me in the eye, and spent a lot of time judging and blaming the people who, he believed, had caused his problems.

Whenever clients have a large investment in diminishing others, I try to discover why they're diminishing themselves. "Steve," I asked, "When did you start feeling this way about these people?"

"About the time I learned that my business partner skipped town, leaving me to repay $300,000 of debt." He didn't sound angry, only defeated.

"And how did you feel about yourself?"

"I failed my family!" he began to sob. "My children, who are in college, are giving money to my wife so we can pay our utility bills."

I let him keep on condemning himself. After a few more minutes, he'd laid out a perfectly justified case.

"Steve," I finally asked, "can you see how your depression and pain are related to the way you're thinking about yourself?"

That got his attention. He was skeptical—the idea flew in the face of all his professional training—but he was interested. Who wouldn't be, after realizing that a variety of medications (including alcohol) weren't helping?

I worked with Steve for several months, helping him alter his beliefs about his life's circumstances. We focused on his judgmental image of himself as a failure. He laughed when I told him about my favorite bumper sticker: *IF YOU CAN'T CHANGE YOUR MIND, YOU DON'T HAVE ONE.*

"These lessons you've undergone," I suggested, "are actually allies that wanted to help you learn the power of thought. Most of us limit ourselves purely by the thoughts we think. Furthermore, at every moment, you and I are determining the power of our thoughts and words. Do you honestly want to believe what you're thinking right now?"

Steve gave me a wry smile. "I *do* have a choice, don't I?"

"Sure you do! Whenever we deny our sacredness and validity, we end up believing we're not deserving—that we have no right to abundance and fulfillment and health. Needless to say, we're always saddened by the result. Could it be your lessons are trying to tell you that you need to get better at the job of loving yourself?"

I assigned him an experiment. ("Exercises" sound too much like work; explorations and experiments are more fun—because you never know what the outcome might be!) For the next week,

Steve was to change any negative self-judgments to thoughts of loving himself. "Even when you hear judgments on television," I grinned, "focus on a thought of loving yourself."

The next time I saw Steve, he was brimming with appreciation. He'd discovered that he did have a choice about what thoughts to "buy," and that he could replace any limiting thought with a more powerful one.

Albert Einstein's breakthrough formula, $E = mc^2$, did wonders for Western thought by demonstrating that energy and physical matter are basically the same thing, and interchangeable. From there, it's no great leap to recognize that our thoughts direct energy.

One night at dinner, I'd been hiccupping for about twenty minutes when my friend Jerry pretended to jab my hand with a fork. For an instant, I was aghast: How could Jerry, of all people, try to stab me? But then I saw he was chuckling—and I, too, roared with laughter when I realized that my hiccups had immediately stopped.

What thoughts are *you* going to entertain? That's an immensely powerful choice! By letting your mind run on automatic, you're deciding to manifest whatever's sitting around in your subconscious memory banks. Which is a little like grabbing whatever's at the back of the refrigerator and serving it for dinner!

Your conscious, outer mind is not who you are. It's merely a tool, to be used as a manifestation-machine, not meant to define, control, or justify the self. Its job is to direct energy. Although it traffics in symbols, you and your experiences inhabit a far larger reality, so vast that those symbols can't begin to contain it.

The outer mind is very proud of itself! When left to its own devices, it thinks its highest purpose is to sit in judgment of every single event that catches our attention. Once a thought occurs, often we start living our lives to justify it. If, at age seven, we're told that fat people are ugly, we'll spend the rest of our lives justifying our dislike of fat people. We'll self-righteously punish fat people—especially if we put on weight ourselves!

Consequently, we've created belief systems that nurture snobbism, prejudice, and bigotry. Simple repetition is all it takes to create a belief system (witness the mega-billion dollar advertising industry I used to be part of!). So, you want to be *very* careful how you let your mind be programmed. Most of us are very unhappy about what our unexamined belief systems are manifesting!

Max Freeman Long, who researched the Hawaiian Huna philosophy early in the twentieth century, was delighted to discover the Huna model for the mind. The ancient Hawaiians believed the conscious mind to be directly connected to the subconscious; and that the subconscious is wired directly to the Higher Self. The subconscious contained all information about one's body, one's personal dimensions, and all the facts and feelings that one has sought to hide and deny. The Higher Self was thought to be unlimited and eternal, holding access to all knowledge and power. So, according to the Huna model, the conscious mind must be able to explore automatic subconscious thinking (e.g., fat people are ugly), and remove self-imposed limitations, in a manner far easier than our conventional wisdom suggests. Can we open the door to the subconscious and make life be an expression of the Unlimited Self?

Since whatever you focus on will manifest sooner or later, why not develop the mental discipline to select thoughts that nurture your *abilities*, which support your greatest desires? One single question will bring this idea down to earth: *If the thought you're thinking right now were to manifest in physical form, would you be pleased?*

Tim was a client who came to me after ten years of frustrating physical and mental limitations, following a stroke. He'd been working hard to recover his motor skills, but despaired that his mental acuity and short-term memory problems would ever return to normal. During one of our sessions, I instructed Tim to close his eyes and focus his awareness on the part of his brain that he thought was damaged. "How does that feel?" I asked.

"It feels dead," he replied, woodenly.

"Okay, Tim. Would you be willing to give up labeling that part of your brain that way?"

He opened his eyes and started to protest: "But every doctor and therapist I've seen for the last ten years—!"

"Fine, Tim, fine," I replied. "For now, let the past go. Just focus on the sensation in that part of your head."

Tim resumed the process. In a few minutes, he began to feel tingling through the whole left side of his brain—and the right side of his body. (As I'm sure you know, the brain's left hemisphere controls the right side of the body, and vice versa.) In the weeks that followed, Tim's progress continued. He reported that much of the mental dysfunction from the stroke was leaving his body— which excited me almost as much as it did him.

How did Tim accomplish this? Simply by giving up a limiting judgment so cruelly powerful that it had severely restricted his life for a full decade. For me, watching him heal himself was like watching a man walk out of prison.

For too long, doctors, diet books, and cancer-awareness postage stamps have warned that your body is an enemy. It is a capricious thing, unwilling to communicate with us, dominated by a mysterious subconscious. It seems to take constant struggle to bring it under control. Health seems to become something for which we must strive and work and pay huge sums of money, rather than our birthright. No wonder we abdicate responsibility for our bodies, turning them over to those more educated, well-paid, and solemn!

Yet our physical bodies are constantly sending us messages for the purpose of restoring health. (And the more we detoxify our bodies of a lifetime of mental and physical toxins, the easier it is to hear the messages our body is sending!) Our pains are telling us we're engaged in a process of healing. When in this process of learning to communicate with the body/subconscious, it's useful to relax, since bodies under stress heal much more slowly.

Next time you feel weary or fatigued, try this experiment: Stop whatever you're doing and simply sit still, with your eyes closed. Locate where in your body the feelings of tiredness reside. Breathe ten deep, connected breaths, focusing on your sensations of fatigue. Listen for the still, quiet voice within. If your conscious mind directs you to get busy and distract yourself, simply direct it to relax, and focus on the sensations of tiredness.

After ten breaths, resume your activity. Notice how your physical experience has changed!

Like Tim, many of my clients deny their own power to heal. Whenever they think they're powerless to overcome imbalances, they resort to the behaviors and attitudes of a victim. To remain in their sympathetic and powerless role, they must remain convinced that they had nothing to do with their plight.

Jayne is a world-class concert pianist. She came to me complaining that her enormous musical talent was only causing her frustration. As a child prodigy, Jayne felt she had been tricked and manipulated into performing. Now she had reached a crossroads: Should she give up the piano entirely and refocus on her troublesome teenagers, or undertake concerts again? She was plagued by fears that any attempt to play music using her own, non-traditional approach would end in failure.

After several sessions, Jayne began to talk about her childhood. Her father had suffered from depression, and her mother considered it her responsibility to make her husband happy. To everyone but Jayne's mom, it was obvious that she was destined to fail. Meanwhile, Jayne was pushed to study piano incessantly and was prodded to perform at public concerts.

Getting back to this present point in her life, she acknowledged that her major struggles revolved around her music and her marriage. "Okay," I said. "Tell me about your relationship with your husband."

"Oh, Rob and I haven't gotten along for years," she replied offhandedly—as if that were the norm for any long-term marriage. "He's always complaining about his failing business, and he never listens to my suggestions that could help."

I decided to go deeper. "Do you see any similarity between how you relate to Rob and how your mom related to your dad?"

Immediately Jayne became agitated. "Yes!" she replied. "We both picked men who don't have the sense to listen to simple advice. It's incredibly frustrating!"

Jayne said she'd always believed that her parents' and teachers' manipulations were the cause of the pain and anger in her relationships. Now, however, we talked about the possibility that she herself, and not her parents or spouse, had created her pain and frustration.

"Jayne," I continued, "do you recognize how you've been blaming others for the choices you made?"

"But I didn't *have* a choice!" she complained.

"Then," I countered, "who ultimately decided that you would play music?"

She hesitated, then suddenly exclaimed, "Oh, I see! I remember being about three years old and deciding that I would play the piano, no matter how unpleasant my mom was. I thought if I played well enough, she'd be nicer to me."

"Suppose your thoughts are actions," I suggested. "Might your life's emotions and circumstances be merely children of the thoughts you choose to think? Your mind is a powerful tool. Distortions in thought," I went on, "produce pain and are the greatest hurdle to accessing the creative power that is your birthright. Why not accept responsibility for how you use that tool? Be willing to change any thought that limits you!"

Jayne saw how she'd blamed herself for her mother's pain: She'd been playing music in an attempt to change her mother's emotions, rather than letting her music express her own heart and soul. Jayne's fears of failure were rooted in the thought that she hadn't succeeded in improving her mother's disposition. Once she finally gave up trying to win her mother's love, Jayne became free to pursue her own unique musical expression—and her concerts have become exciting for her, and rewarding for her audience. Also, courageously, she began dropping her blame of Rob and found her marriage improving as well.

Too many of my clients believe that their thoughts make no difference at all—an apparently innocent belief system that's the source of most of the limitations they experience in life!

When he was a boy, Randall believed he was unlovable. He justified that point of view with the humiliation he felt when his alcoholic father seemed to favor his brothers over him—and when they teased him. So as Randall grew up, he began treating himself as if he were truly unlovable, soon forgetting that this decision was self-imposed.

By the time Randall and I began working together, he'd amassed a string of failed relationships—with women and employers. The females kept telling him he was too manipulative, and his employers warned that he wasn't a team player. Very soon, Randall discovered his basic operating principle: Convincing others that he was lovable. Rather than granting others the choice to love him or not, he took on the enormous and never-ending task of making *everybody* love Randall.

In one of our sessions, he was understandably stunned to recall a day decades ago, in his early childhood, when he decided he was simply unlovable. Ever since, Randall's life had been one long, accurate reflection of that subconsciously held belief—and its terrible power!

Tara came to work with me because she had been troubled for years with loneliness. "Why do I always find myself with men who aren't emotionally available?" she complained. Later on, during that first session, she recognized that she was hiding from her own fear of loneliness by putting herself into relationships that she didn't really want. As we began to explore more deeply, Tara discovered that she had been using her fear of loneliness to avoid the deeper childhood pain of feeling unlovable—which, she believed, meant that she really *was* unlovable! In accepting her sensations of fear,

Tara was able to heal the pain of feeling unlovable, and no longer keep it as a belief about herself.

Whenever a painful emotion or chronic physical condition persists, it helps to explore your thinking. Often my clients block the healing process with counterproductive beliefs and limiting attitudes. One of the most persistent (and effective!) doubts that they cling to is, "I really don't have the power to heal." Variations on this theme include:

"This pain is too serious to heal."

"I blame someone else for this pain, so first, I must get revenge."

"Before I can heal, I must be punished."

"I don't deserve to be healed."

"I can't commit to healing myself."

"I don't have God's permission."

To many of us, healing processes seem alien and unknown, so of course we fear to begin them. Yet we can learn to heal even our fear of healing, and begin to attain peace with our bodies. We can learn to trust our powers to heal, express our uniqueness, and create our own unique gifts for this world.

Healing is a birthright, natural to every living creature. Put another way, if we have the power to create an imbalance, we must have the inherent ability to restore that balance. And it takes far *less* energy to heal an imbalance than it took to create it.

There's no great magic in claiming our power to heal. The work is in discovering how we've impeded our own healing processes. Healing accesses greater energy, while creating imbalance drains energy. Thus, if your life isn't reflecting what you want to create, it pays to uncover the ways you're using energy to create blocks.

Journal Exploration #1

Removing Blocks

1. Quiet yourself. Breathe. Now, list three persistent conflicts, pains, or limitations that you have trouble healing.

2. If these situations were to vanish from your life, what's the worst-case scenario that could occur? Are you willing to accept that?

3. List three conflicts, pains, or limitations that you don't deserve to have healed—or for which you blame others.

4. What would convince you that you deserve to be healed?

5. Are you willing to forgive yourself? What do you need before you can forgive others?

Frank thought he'd failed his son by being a strict, controlling father during Mike's developmental years. He didn't realize that these judgmental thoughts had been producing his guilt feelings. I picked up on this after Frank kept defending himself whenever he talked about Mike's distance. To Frank, it seemed perfectly sensible to blame himself for Mike's decisions. That also kept him trying to compensate for the past—which his son naturally found distasteful.

On the day we finally touched on the belief that he'd been a bad father, Frank exclaimed, "Yeah, I guess I am hardest on myself!" That set him on the path to forgiving himself and being more honest in his communications with his son.

Realizing how powerful our thoughts are helps us to remember to choose them consciously. When my clients are learning this, I often tell them that the ancient Essenes offered a prayer to the Angel of Power: "Make my thoughts stronger than death."

Experiment #2

Re-Training the Rational Mind

Under stress? Take a moment and just breathe. Listen to your mind. Focus on the thought you're thinking.

A thought of diminishment, is it? What if that worry were going to manifest in three minutes? Would you want to keep on thinking it? If not, then gently tell your rational mind to replace that thought with one that's powerful and supportive—for example, "I am an unlimited child of the universe!"

Then go on with your day. Every time a diminishing thought occurs, replace it with the new one—that you're *un*limited.

Simply repeating the new thought will eventually stimulate your rational mind to start justifying it. The mind is meant to be re-programmed whenever it's obvious that we've outgrown the existing programming— and we have, in spades!

Thoughts are actions, and powerful ones at that. During a firewalking workshop, I told the students that their focus had everything to do with their experience of walking safely across over-

800-degree coals. One woman walked the fire several times, quite safely. Then, back home, she told her friends and coworkers of her experience. She heard (and obviously believed) so many of their skeptical opinions that three days later, blisters appeared on her feet.

Energy follows focus; energy follows thought. Put another way, the abundant energy pervading this universe is simply awaiting your direction to begin moving toward physical manifestation. Thought is a very powerful tool to get that energy flowing.

Experiment #5

The Power of Focus in Creating Reality

Next time you're carrying a bag of groceries, stop and pay attention. Where do you experience the bag's weight? Probably you'll feel the weight a few inches above your hand, somewhere in the center of the bag.

Now, visualize the weight as levitating about twelve to eighteen inches *above* the bag.

Maintain that focus. Is carrying the groceries easier or harder? Can you carry the groceries farther than you could otherwise?

Create your own variations on this experiment with any physical exertion.

(*Helpful hint: Breathing helps!*)

~ ~ ~

In the healing support groups I lead, one requirement is that participants arrive on time. During the early years with the groups, students would sometimes call me on their cell phones: "Ned, the traffic is backed up; we're going to be delayed." I'd gently chastise these people for not leaving home early enough. But the problem persisted.

Then I began taking a different tack: "Thanks for your call. I suggest that you focus on the slowed or stalled cars ahead. Visualize them flowing smoothly, like a river of white light. Maintain this image until the traffic moves. Whenever your mind intrudes with a judgment or distraction, simply push the thought aside and gently refocus on the river of white light, flowing to my office."

This gave them something to focus on while waiting. With a little practice, they could effectively support a smooth flow of traffic. Before long, these people began arriving on time—even when they'd called to warn me they'd be late! These students taught other participants about imagining a river of white light—and now, I very rarely get such calls!

Experiment #7

Demonstrating the Power of Focus

1. While watching a bird fly through the air, focus on its path. Imagine it slowing down. Continue this experiment until you *experience* the bird slowing down.

2. As a variation on this exercise, cast your gaze on a river. Consciously focus on slowing the river down—then speed it up! After some practice, you can experiment with slowing and speeding the flow of time.

3. Okay, why not? Next time you find yourself in a traffic jam, take a long look at the slowing or stalled cars ahead.

   Visualize them flowing smoothly, like a river of white light, flowing to your destination. Maintain this image until the traffic moves. Whenever your rational mind intrudes with a judgment or distraction, simply push the thought aside. Gently refocus on the river of white light.

   Important note: This tool isn't about using your mind to control other drivers. It's about focusing on what you want—for others' benefit, as well as yours (more on this concept in Chapter 13). If nothing else, this should prompt a dramatic shift in your thoughts, especially when you're stuck in traffic and are questioning *other drivers' immediate ancestry.*

Sometimes, I think of my clients and myself as birds in a darkened room, flying toward lighted windows, willing to keep hitting our heads on the glass until we find an open door. Meanwhile, of course, we've mastered the ability to cower in dark corners, convincing ourselves that we're really comfortable!

I'll suggest a further experiment: By making a few changes in how you relate to the universe's energy, can you turn your life into a powerful, joyful pursuit?

To perform this experiment, you must consider yourself as more than your mind. More than your emotions, physical body, job, image and reputation! These are all *possessions*, which you simply use to express yourself. You—the *real* you—are far greater than that. (*For more on this dynamic concept, see Chapter 10.*)

For now, let me be blunt: You and I are the Creators of our special, personal experiences of the world. Apply this idea to your personal life, and evaluate the results—in line with your own values and priorities.

CHAPTER FOUR

Choices and Commitments

Brad is a professor at a local naturopathic college. "I don't know what I truly want to do with my life," he announced in my office. He described himself as having been a "happy, talkative child," although he was angry with his parents for "telling me to shut up."

As Brad talked about his boyhood, he made it clear how devoted he was to his father. "His eyes would twinkle at me when I was a boy!" he exclaimed. His father's health declined, however, and as Brad reached adulthood he heard his father say, "I don't know what happened to you. You were such a nice kid." Despite six proposals from women, Brad never married, believing he could never get relationships right.

As we talked, Brad came to see how the choices he'd made about himself, based on his parents' beliefs, had become the structure of his life. His ultimate concern was to get his father's eyes to twinkle again. As we worked, Brad sadly found out he could not create happiness in anyone else, much less his father. Instead, he began to explore the ideas that he secretly carried about having fun singing and expressing himself. And over time, Brad recovered his ability to find direction in his life.

Your conscious mind receives a steady stream of messages. The challenge, of course, is to distinguish the ones that reflect a loving universe, from those generated by your outer, rational mind, trying to protect you from unseen, imagined enemies.

Listen carefully, and what do you hear? "Limitation" or "Freedom"?

Many of my clients grew up under strict parenting. Early in life, they decided it simply wasn't safe to make choices freely, that their power to choose was non-existent or simply irrelevant. Trapped in such limited beliefs, they assumed that their desires were pointless; they could not see themselves as powerful beings, and didn't believe they were able to change and grow. They'd forgotten that of all the thoughts drifting through their consciousness, they have a choice over which ones they'll accept, buy into, and believe. (When you go to a seafood restaurant, do you order every lobster in the tank?)

Many of us hesitate to make choices, out of fear of making a mistake. We believe we're not free to express our wants, our point of view, or to simply say "No." But free will is our birthright, integral to our divine essence. We can evolve joyfully, or stagnate— painfully! But your unique validity, and mine, can't be compromised by any of the lessons we take on. We're here to discover ever-larger expressions of our godhood, *without* the need to prove it.

I think it helps to make a distinction between *choices* and *decisions*. Choices are expressions of wants and desires—that is, acts of will, selections made freely. Decisions reflect reasoning, mental evaluation, and judgment. While driving a car, I constantly make *decisions* about obeying the speed limit and stopping for red lights, but *choices* about where I'm going. Our choices seem to be reflections of our uniqueness, our power and energy.

Yes, we must accept the consequences of our actions, but I don't believe that God thinks any less of us for any self-limiting choice; or that our innate innocence and sanctity can be diminished by any choice we make.

Journal Exploration #9

Freedom to Choose

1. In what areas of your life do you feel trapped? (For example, "I'll never have a job that I'll enjoy.")

2. What limiting beliefs do you hold about those areas of life? ("I'm not talented enough to experience prosperity.")

3. What thoughts could you cultivate to fully claim your freedom to choose—under all circumstances? ("My contributions fully express my love for the world.")

Years ago, when I was studying with George, I agreed to present a stress-management program to several of his clients. I was excited and began the project with a vengeance. Yet as the days passed, my excitement waned. I began to fear that the program wasn't all that it was cracked up to be.

After a week of chastising myself, I finally admitted, "I'm having difficulty honoring this commitment, because I no longer feel excited about it."

"Perhaps it's appropriate that your excitement has flagged," George suggested. "Perhaps it's delivered its message and moved on!" He went on to suggest that something else might replace excitement to help me in completing the project.

When I explored what message my initial excitement had left, I realized that I'd needed it to begin the project. Now that I had committed myself, excitement was no longer necessary. Once I accepted that fact, I found an ample supply of enthusiasm and energy to complete the program successfully!

The German philosopher Johann Wolfgang von Goethe wrote: "the moment one definitely commits oneself, then Providence moves too. All sorts of things occur to help that would never have otherwise occurred. A whole stream of events issues from the decision, raising in one's favor all manner of unforeseen incidents and meetings and material assistance which no man could have dreamed would have come his way."

Goethe was saying that energy follows our choices, our thoughts and our focus. Choice and commitment are tools that help us learn the full measure of our power. Within the power of choice—as George helped me discover for myself—lies all the emotional energy you'll need for a favorable outcome.

This is why avoiding commitment and denying your power to choose means condemning yourself to impotence and frustration. Sometimes people ask me, "If I give up my judgments, how am I going to determine my choices?" We've forgotten that our wants and desires are expressions of our deepest passions, rather than the consolation prize after we've discarded everything that we don't want. What would it take to pursue what you truly want and nurture your freedom to choose as well?

The power to commit is the power to create!

To use the abundant, creative energy around us, you must treat your word as the most sacred ability you own. If you make promises haphazardly and make a habit of excuses, this book will have little value for you. Realize that your words are powerful, containing great energy that activates the process of creation. To undertake this journey, you must honor your commitments!

Say that you've promised to deliver a letter for a friend. Then, *deliver the letter!* Even if you've created a sudden debilitating illness and are on your deathbed, see to it that the letter gets delivered. Have you failed at keeping your word? Make amends—and surrender the need to invalidate yourself. If you must renegotiate an agreement, do so in such a way that both parties wind up winning.

Alternate Experiment #11

Facing Procrastination

Assuming you're facing a project you've been putting off, stop! Before you tackle it again, try this.

1. Sit quietly. Close your eyes and breathe. Spend a moment identifying the goal of the project. Focus on any emotional or physical sensations (such as fear of failure). Let yourself breathe deeply and repeatedly as you focus on feeling the sensations.

2. After identifying the feeling that surrounds this procrastination, visualize the project as completed, with these feelings a component of that completion.

3. Immediately following Step #2, perform some concrete action—no matter how small—to move the project forward. Drop any need to judge the result. Commit to the next time you will do more to advance the project.

    Regardless of what may interrupt that commitment, make sure that you complete it on time!

4. Bless yourself.

5. Give thanks for the challenges and learning that the project is bringing into your life.

Here's a secret that it pays to remember: Commitment *always* evokes resistance! Whenever I give someone my word, soon there comes a time when I wish I hadn't, when I doubt the value and wisdom of having done so.

I wasted many years giving up on my commitments, only to discover that doing so didn't serve my growth. Now, I continue to fulfill my word, *especially* when I don't want to or don't feel like it. This has taught me:

1) Never to commit to anything that I won't go that extra mile to complete;

2) That others have every right to demand that I keep my word with them;

3) That I, too, have the right to demand that others honor their agreements with me;

4) Further, that they respect my right to validate myself, to hold myself inviolate.

You have these rights, too! Yet many people refuse to claim them, despite the tremendous power they contain.

In our frantic world, often we try to defer responsibility, rather than own up to our commitments. We become defensive when discussing broken agreements. I've watched myself revert to being a 6-year-old to justify not keeping my word. But whenever I adopt this defensive posture, I'm not letting myself be honest about my feelings of guilt, failure, shame, and disappointment. Thus, I'm unable to heal that pain and learn from the experience. I'm destined to repeat the failed commitment, sometime in the future!

Whenever you and I sell out our integrity and don't clean up our messes, it costs us our freedom to love and validate ourselves. It costs us our access to our unlimited power and potential. A very useful experiment is to make a list of the top ten commitments you've not honored, and then move those broken agreements to completion, a place where you are at peace with them.

When our commitments don't seem to unfold the way we've asked, could it be that we've shaped a commitment to avoid feeling some pain, loss or guilt? Perhaps we've manifested a subconscious belief that's impeding what we truly want. I once asked for a new romance, only to face a long period of solitude. When I finally got honest about my experience, I had to face a pit of loneliness that I was desperate to avoid. From that, I learned that the loneliness was a messenger, not a permanent condition. This lesson helped me use the energy of my commitments to accept the validity of all my experiences, not just those that fit my expectations. Imagine the experience of feeling unworthiness, guilt, and shame as messengers seeking to support the growth of your abilities!

Completing commitments is a powerful way of accessing more creative energy. Whenever we acknowledge ourselves (or another) for fulfilling a commitment, we actually propel ourselves into a new level of growth. Completing commitments isn't about boasting, it's about release. So, telling your friend that you've delivered the letter fulfills your responsibility, and allows that energy to recycle on to your next project. Honoring our own commitments could be a great step in reclaiming our validity and accessing our tremendous power to heal and create. Perhaps we each were meant to commit to honoring our own unique validity!

Experiment #12

Nurturing your Validity

1. First thing in the morning, stand in front of a mirror. Look yourself straight in the eyes.

2. Say out loud, "I alone am responsible for my worth. Under all circumstances, I can be counted on to honor my own validity."

3. Repeat this declaration three times, while breathing deeply and accepting your feelings. Maintain eye contact with your mirror image.

4. Do this exercise every day for twenty-one days.

5. Give thanks.

Be prepared to trust yourself more and more. (When you were an infant, you couldn't trust yourself to walk—yet today, you can!) Don't be surprised if you lose the need to justify your experience. Let every choice reveal your unique magnificence, rather than the need to prove it!

Whenever your rational mind questions the validity of your experience, change that thought! Continue to change those invalidating thoughts, until your mind adopts the new way of thinking.

Many people assume that cynicism—doubting themselves and the world around them—is a sign of intelligence and sophistication. Yet rarely do those fashionable doubters consider the wisdom of doubting their own doubts!

Experiment #13

Checked Your Doubts Lately?

1. Spend one day watching for thoughts devoted to doubt. Upon becoming aware of a doubt, simply note it. At the end of the day, rate your satisfaction with your quality of life—during this one 24-hour period-— on a scale of 1 to 10.

2. The next day, consciously focus on questioning your doubts. Again, rate the quality of your life on a scale of 1 to 10.

3. On succeeding days, you choose! Does doubting your doubts improve your quality of life?

Chapter Five
Where to Start: the Sacred Present

A number of my clients complain of a feeling of heaviness across their torso. When I help them explore that sensation, invariably they discover they've constructed a shield to protect themselves from rejection or disappointment. "You needn't protect yourself from your own experiences," I tell them. "Validate them and let them support your growth."

How easily we abdicate the present, and focus on the past and future! But only in the present can we truly feel—with all our senses, with total awareness and complete attention. And so, given humankind's vast commitment to divorcing itself from the present, we have yet to evolve past being controlled by our emotions and our feelings.

At times when I'm upset or in pain, someone will ask, "How are you, Ned?" and I will lie and answer, "I'm fine." Yet whenever I'm not able to accept whatever pain I'm feeling right here, right now, I manage to block my ability to heal that same pain.

Quite unknowingly, the energy of denial creates many limitations. Hiding our present experience in the folds of the subconscious not only takes energy, but it also stops growth and healing. And the problem will have to be faced sooner or later, only adding to our anguish.

A client, Judy, told me about her debilitating fear of being ridiculed. When we began exploring more deeply, she related the story of a day in kindergarten, when here classmates were laughing at her. Her teacher admonished her, "Don't cry, Judy. Why don't you feed the goldfish instead?" Even at five years old, Judy knew feeding goldfish didn't heal pain, but she complied to avoid more ridicule from the class. Judy learned how to give up avoiding that sensation, and accept her power to feel it—and heal it.

To access your power to heal, you must be focused in the present, not on the past when the pain first began; not on some future time when it will be cured. Thus, you must be willing to accept your pains *now*, and suspend any negative beliefs about them. (*More about this in Chapter 7!*)

As you undertake this book, stop invalidating your so-called failings, addictions, and weaknesses. *Do not diminish the validity of your experience, ever!*

Journal Exploration #13

Accepting the Truth of your Experience

1. List the feelings that you were hiding today. (Extra credit for seeing those you hid from yourself!)

2. After identifying those hidden feelings, ask yourself, "During the moment of my denial, what was it I truly wanted?"

With the advent of mass media, we're able to imagine future scenarios with great ease. *However, we weren't given imaginations to invalidate the present moment!* Often we never realize we've gone "future shopping," looking at possible predictions, then relating and reacting to those events as if they were real in the here-and-now. Often we deny our present pain, hoping that our future-shopping trip will be successful.

I came to understand this distortion when Marie, a very wealthy woman, came to see me, seeking to rid herself of deep fears and anxieties in her life. In our sessions together, she discovered that she was depending on wealth to protect her from her worst-case scenario: seeing herself as a bag lady!

Since then, Marie has learned that she's not powerless over the future; that she can manifest whatever she truly wants. Now, rather than believing in any "future shopping" predictions, she trusts that her power—her ability to focus her creative awareness—lies in the present.

Like Marie, at times I seek to avoid worst-case scenarios, rather than focus on what I truly have, right here and now. Choosing to accept the present lets me gain direct access to manifesting what I truly want—in fact, that's the only way to do it! Here's a motto to tattoo on your grey cells:

> The Present is
> the Only
> Point of Power.

The present is the only "place" where you can create, heal, love and connect with your unlimited, eternal Self. It's the only moment when God is available. It's the only time you can exercise your powerful relationship with energy.

Every instant gives you a new opportunity to focus awareness—into acceptance or resistance. This present moment is always an answer to your thoughts, choices and prayers. The present—right now—is the only time you can make a choice! *Right now is the only time when you can make any choice at all!*

Can you give up being suspicious of the present moment? Imagine that this present instant is the best manifestation you could possibly create to support human evolution. In other words, give up debating the validity of yourself and whatever's happening now!

Play with the concept that every succeeding instant is the universe's best effort to communicate!

Not clear whether you're fully in the present? Simply stop, and breathe! Focus within! Simply feel whatever sensations are occurring in your body—like the weight of this book in your hand, the pages between your fingers. Take time to become aware of the specific components of your present experience.

Connected Breathing

Every so often, exploring these ideas will very likely require a pause for integration. At such times, I recommend taking long, deep, consciously connected breaths.

Every culture that developed effective healing techniques has embraced breathing as a core tool for restoring balance. Breath not only oxygenates the blood, but also restores its acid/alkaline pH balance. Therapists use it to help clients release toxins more effectively; and you'll find that connected breathing is a wondrous tool to help you release mental toxins as well!

To do so, completely fill your lungs. Gradually release that breath. Then, upon emptying your lungs, connect with the next full inhalation.

Experiment by taking three connected breaths now.

Breath is your ally in helping you connect with the power in the present. Notice how this helps you connect with being in your body—which is imperative for the effective use of energy! Whenever I'm facing a stressful situation, I begin by taking ten connected breaths.

Throughout this book, watch for the breathing symbol:

~ ~ ~

—as a signal to connect yourself with the Sacred Present. You'll find that connected breathing helps you integrate information and speeds growth and healing. This single exercise alone can transform your life!

One reason (and there are plenty!) why we created this dimension collectively, is to learn to trust ourselves *individually*— validate our unique experiences, and enjoy the oneness underlying all relationships. Learning to trust the present moment, you trust the power available at *every* moment, as well as your unique God within.

Trust the power of breathing! That's part of the lesson!

~ ~ ~

One of my clients complained, "If I stop trying to resist what I hate in the present moment, won't I be powerless to change it?" I told her that for accessing power, accepting the present is a must. We're never free to create as long as we're resisting, judging, bellyaching, or attempting any form of control. We've become very skilled at a multitude of expressions of resistance, yet it only causes us to get stuck in whatever experience we're resisting. It stops growth, and causes stagnation, a condition many of us don't even realize we're mired in!

Ron, the manager of a local bank, came to see me, feeling disappointed and overwhelmed. He was at the top of his profession, but his position as manager required many overtime hours. His children felt neglected and his wife was threatening to leave. Ron was using his failures at home as justification for diminishing himself. But as you can imagine, this stress cycled back into his working hours at the bank, creating even more difficulties to overcome.

Over several sessions, we worked through the Heal-a-Hurt

Exercise (*see page 72*), focusing first on Ron's feeling overwhelmed. He discovered that he could, indeed, face these challenges.

Next, we focused on his disappointment. Ron realized he wasn't pursuing what was truly important to him. He'd been substituting success for love and felt imprisoned in his life. The more he learned to accept his current emotions, the more Ron allowed himself to pursue what meant the most in life—the love he felt for his wife and children.

Investing more time and attention with his family ultimately improved Ron's performance at work. Accepting his present discomfort let him connect with the joy that was *also* readily available in his life. In accepting his pain, Ron learned that he'd been resisting facing the risk of pursuing what he truly wanted.

We have the great power to choose to accept or resist any experience. All too often, we resist our painful experiences, simply because we don't like them, losing sight of the fact that pain is integral to the healing process. We must heal in order to grow— the only direction life moves in. Not to worry, however, for if you find yourself growing at a breakneck pace, simply resist where you are, and you'll come to a screeching halt. Pain is simply the universe's way of telling us we've become too dependent on staying stuck. Acceptance always accesses growth, and our growth can always be trusted!

Living in the present teaches you to give up dependence and claim the truth of your own power. When you accept whatever shows up in the Sacred Present, you discover that each current event is exactly what you need to grow toward—and ultimately, create—what you truly desire (*as you'll see in Chapter 13*)!

PART TWO

Healing Yourself

CHAPTER SIX
Don't Shoot the Messenger!

From Pain to Healing

I have frequent opportunities to teach seminars. At one called "Reclaiming the Power to Heal," a woman asked, "Why did we—with God's help—create a universe where pain exists? Is it to punish us?"

"If punishment nurtured growth," I replied, "we'd have saints walking out of prisons!"

Just how young were you, when you first decided that pain was bad? From that, you deduced and decreed, "Whenever I'm in pain, I'm being punished. That means I'm wrong. Pain proves that I've failed."

Many of us measure our success by how well we avoid pain. I think we've lost sight of the value of growth and replaced it with the idea of comfort; losing our ability to learn from pain—which I define as any of the spectrum of sensations that we simply don't like. Many of us have come to believe that we can't heal pain; that it's bigger than we are!

Countless medical studies have shown that denying and repressing emotional pain leads to stress, high blood pressure, immune dysfunction and disease, including cancer. Worse, mistrusting pain means ignoring one of life's quickest routes to the expansion of further growth, power and freedom.

By "learning from pain," I don't mean trial and error. I mean directly. We have a natural ability to communicate with pain— and experience the healing that occurs automatically as soon as we understand its message. Pain is simply a messenger, telling us there is some distortion in our thoughts. It's telling us that we've focused on a lie. Once we get its message, the messenger moves on. We call this healing—our natural birthright.

Try an experiment! For one week, assume that pain is neither good nor bad, but only a messenger trying to alert you to distortions in your thinking—pointing out where you're using your own thoughts to limit yourself.

Journal Exploration #15

1. What were your family's unspoken rules for dealing with pain? (Blame, justification, distraction, anger, avoidance?)

2. What thoughts do you use to avoid your feelings? ("I'm too busy right now." "Others need me." "People would feel uncomfortable if I were emotionally honest." "I shouldn't feel this way.")

3. When you're in pain, what do you believe about yourself? ("I'm weak." "I'm unworthy." "God's punishing me.")

Several months after my father died, I visited his home to collect some mementos of our shared experiences. Alone there, as I selected a few ties and accessories, I found it surprising that I didn't feel any grief or sadness.

I packed up and drove to the airport. My flight's departure time was fast approaching, but the rental car agency was very gracious and accommodating. As I hurried from their office, I saw their driver waiting for me, holding open the door to the van.

As I launched my body through the door, I neglected to duck and cracked the crown of my head soundly against the doorjamb.

After literally seeing stars, my first thought was that I wouldn't have hit my head if the driver hadn't been holding the door. Then—realizing that was stretching blame pretty far! —I decided to see if the pain had any message for me. I began deep, connected breathing and focused on the sensation. Yes, it hurt, but I just accepted the discomfort rather than trying to manage it. When I asked the pain if there was any message, I immediately heard, *You're in pain.* I realized the message was about my hidden grief over my father's death— and not the bump on my head.

By itself, this was no great revelation. But when I realized that I'd invested considerable energy in denying my grief throughout the whole trip, the severe pain at the top of my head disappeared—immediately!

Several minutes afterwards, I opened up to the feelings of fear and loss, loneliness and isolation that I'd been avoiding. Then, over the next several days, I was able to accept those emotions and the messages they carried—which helped me confront deep fears about my own mortality.

This example illustrates the radical idea that when dealing with pain, acceptance is much more powerful than resistance.

Take a look at your personal universe, and you'll see that growth is the natural direction of things. Life is inherently designed to express joy and fulfillment. But when we make choices based on misconception and denial, the universe lets us know it. By the time pain finally shows up, we've spent enormous energy on distortions, ignoring the many subtle physical, mental and emotional signals that are meant to correct the lies we believe.

The real problem is, we don't view pain as integral to the healing process. When in pain, we judge ourselves as unhealthy, and we block pain's messages with negative self-judgment:"Since I'm feeling bad, I must be unworthy. I must deserve to be punished."

This kind of self-diminishment simply blocks healing. Too often, we become masters at distracting ourselves from pain by drinking, drugging, and having sex. We've come to depend on our TVs, VCRs and petty squabbles to take our attention off our hurting. As a result, we grow increasingly addicted to things which are supposed to make us happy (but don't!). Meanwhile, mired in pain and unhappiness, we adopt a lifestyle of blaming, judging, and controlling others. We're stuck and trying to prove we're happy about that!

All too often—as in certain therapies—we attempt to *understand* our pain, at the cost of our willingness to feel it. Thus, energy held within pain is stagnant, and not allowed to flow. So, here are some nasty misconceptions you must avoid: *Pain is not punishment. It's not payback for your sins. Pain is not God's way of telling you that you're bad!*

~ ~ ~

One of my clients believed that every time her body hurt, it had betrayed her. Another believed that every time he felt pain, it meant he was separate from God. Whenever someone close to him fell ill, his grandfather would demand,"Who in this family is living wrong?"

Pain is like the earsplitting noise of a smoke detector—not at all pleasant, but guaranteed to get your attention. Pain is only prompting us to examine our focus, our thoughts. Pain is merely our way of teaching ourselves to claim ownership of our choices and to discover those choices that impede our own growth. Once we get the message, the messenger can move on—and we experience healing. And in the process, we learn to love ourselves, even when in pain!

Greg was his mother's favorite child. As a youngster, he felt guilty about this, especially when he saw his older brother, Tom, receiving less attention. Greg decided to love Tom more as a way of atoning. During his sessions with me, Greg started facing his guilt and, as it healed, he discovered why his relationship with his brother hadn't worked. His guilt gave him the message that love must be a choice, never an obligation—and Greg recovered his freedom to love Tom, to be honest, and to love himself in the process!

This example demonstrates the common, but totally unworkable, misperception that holding onto pain can help us serve and love others. Martyrdom isn't healing, it's control.

Another misconception is that pain is to be feared. Instead of simply accepting this fear, learning from pain, and letting it depart in peace; we try to avoid, control, and protect ourselves—which also blocks healing.

Our relationship with pain is mirrored in all our other relationships—and it shapes them, as well. Because we think it is to be feared, we close off our ability to feel, to desire, to access our passion for living. As a result, many of my clients feel "dead"— sorry gruel indeed, compared to the liveliness that our addictions can never replace.

Pain has never been our enemy, but our ally for healing, once we learn how to communicate with it effectively. For centuries, we've been brainwashed into thinking that healing is an ability restricted to saints and duly certified physicians. Many of us have been taught that we must die before we can fully heal. No wonder my clients are so surprised when they discover that they can indeed heal themselves!

~ ~ ~

My client Jean was working her way through painful memories of an abusive childhood. One day, as I was guiding her toward her feelings of anxiety, she connected with herself as a three-year-old girl playing with matches. Her father caught her at it and spanked her.

Surprised to remember the humiliation of the experience, Jean saw how her three-year-old self had made a decision: "This pain is too big. I don't have the power to heal it. I'll just have to carry it around for the rest of my life." Jean's anxiety told her that, in fact, her father wasn't to blame for her humiliation—but her own beliefs were.

You'll never have a discomfort that's beyond your ability to heal!

Every feeling, pleasant or not, has a beginning and an end. If you can just accept and feel your present sensation for its duration, you'll find it very simple to get the message. If your pain seems to be stuck, explore and see if you're blaming someone else for it. Blame always blocks healing.

Does pain hurt? Darn right! But the time it takes you to heal it is brief. (After a little practice, you'll need only a few moments!) And healing completes the process of getting the message, forestalling a lifetime of denial. The pain won't continue to plague you, contributing to unwanted behaviors, addictions and obsessions that often seem unmanageable.

Healing is not a reward you've earned, it's your birthright!!

Acceptance leads to growth and healing. Resistance merely stretches your baggage-handling capacity. The universe (doing business as Reality) is always moving in the direction of growth. So why not go with the flow?

Here's how you go about it: The first step is to breathe fully. For the moment, suspend the idea that pain's purpose is to damage or punish you. (I often joke that the primary message of any discomfort is, "Suspend your mental analyzing!") Accept the sensation as a messenger, not as an enemy.

Accept whatever pain you face in this moment. Continue to breathe.

~ ~ ~

Stop *thinking* about pain, and simply *feel* it. Locate the sensation in your body. This messenger speaks in the language of sensation, and its healing message points to your own profound uniqueness and the gifts you have to offer to this world. (*For more on that topic, see Chapter 13!*)

Some of my clients worry, "Won't giving in to pain—or any other unpleasant reality— rob me of my self-control? Doesn't that mean surrendering my freedom of choice?"

Not so! By accepting pain, you're *more* able to interact with your body and your present circumstances, *more* able to express yourself fully and honestly. Acknowledging and allowing whatever is, lets you relate to the present, where you're able to listen and access your power of choice.

Once you've allowed the sensation, then ask if there's a message. Focus on listening, not deducing. Give up on expecting or predicting a message. Simply be receptive to whatever comes into your consciousness. (This trains your rational mind to be receptive as well as expressive—to be your servant rather than your master.)

As you listen, be open to the pain revealing a belief in limitation, a belief you've really believed is true—

~~~

—and see if a process of growth doesn't begin automatically.

Explore any belief that denies you the freedom to make your own choices, for this is the source of much of our pain today.

Are There Other Messages on The Tape?

To make the necessary choices that nurture healing, you must bring pain to consciousness—you must stop hiding it.

Do you suspect you might be in denial? Just ask to have the hidden pain revealed. Yep, it's that easy! If you prefer to direct the request in a specific direction, ask your body (or your cells, your subconscious, your dreams, or your Higher Power) to show you what you've hidden from yourself.

Ask that all that is unseen become seen. Remember to give thanks for the result, at the time of asking.

After you've asked, breathing is a good thing.

~ ~ ~

Asking for what you want (*as you'll see in Chapter 11*) releases energy to work for you. Don't worry about when you'll receive an answer, just hold yourself receptive. Sometimes I get the message when I'm casually driving the car, or taking a shower—when my mind isn't actively engaged.

Very often, you'll create some event that dramatizes whatever you're holding in denial. How can that be? Well, the universe is designed to support your growth and greatest fulfillment. It wants you to be free of your self-imposed limitations. We were never meant to manage our own growth, but all too often that's what our controlling behaviors are about. Try simply asking for growth and then accepting whatever shows up as its expression. Growth should be joyfully and easily available in everyday life!

Looking into your denials is one of the greatest expressions of loving yourself. Love will bring up anything unlike itself to be healed, so make sure you're ready to receive the response.

Once you're clear about your avoidance mechanisms, experiment with accepting your pain. Doesn't that choice serve you better than resistance?

Often we deny pain because allowing it might evoke conflict with someone else. Other times we hide our feelings, for fear of violating our cherished self-image. We may believe that denial is the noble "stiff upper lip" way of reacting to pain, thereby not annoying or distressing our loved ones. But asking others to explore their own denials is a powerful way to access energy in our relationships. This requires that we be honest with each other and willing to gently explore our hiding places, without judgment. It means that we're willing to deliver uncomfortable messages to each other, without compromising our willingness to love.

Happiness doesn't mean that we'll never feel pain. Give up that expectation! Can we build relationships that permit us to ask one another about our pain and our denials?

Whenever my clients start taking responsibility for their pain, invariably they go through a period of intensified emotion, during which they deal with whatever pain they've been resisting. Once through this process, however, they become aware of subtler feelings and insights, which can heal the deeper core distortions in their lives and open doors to deeper dimensions of the self.

True healing always addresses the underlying source of an imbalance, be it mental, physical or emotional. True healing must correct the underlying way you're using energy to produce the distortion. Therefore, you must be able to move from the symptom (often physical) to the cause (conscious or subconscious). All healing is multidimensional, moving you to where you can create your experience, and expand your consciousness at the same time.

Experiment #17

Heal A Hurt

1. Locate the pain.

2. Begin breathing deeply, connecting your breaths, throughout the exercise.

   ~ ~ ~

3. Tell your mind to go to the beach! This is feeling time, not problem-solving, analyzing or fixing-it time.

   ~ ~ ~

4. Get sensual. Let your body experience the pain in its specific location.

   ~ ~ ~

5. How does the sensation feel, warm or cool? What's its texture, rough or sharp? How heavy does it feel? Keep breathing.

   ~ ~ ~

6. Give yourself permission to feel this pain. Let your body feel it. Allow the pain to be there, just as it is.

   Give up any need to oppose it. (Remind your mind about the beach.)

   ~ ~ ~

7. Move your awareness inside the feeling. Does it feel more like liquid, more dense, or more open? Gently feel through the interior of the pain. (Don't force your way through!) Notice if there's any temperature on the inside, as well. Remain sensual. Keep breathing.

~ ~ ~

8. Notice that you can feel more dimensions of the sensation than you could at first.

~ ~ ~

9. After you've felt all the way through the pain, are you willing to love yourself while you feel it? Then see if you are you willing to let it love you? (You don't know *how* it's going to love you, of course. The question is, are you willing to let in whatever love it may hold?)

~ ~ ~

10. If you're unwilling, end the exercise. (Don't worry, the pain will be back!)

~ ~ ~

11. If you are willing, just tell the pain so, mentally. Then open your body and your cells to being loved. Let in the feeling! Keep breathing.

~ ~ ~

12. After feeling this love, ask if it has a message for you. The message may be another sensation, a memory, a picture, an idea. Your body may simply have wanted you to focus on that spot for a while. How do you know if you got the message? The pain clears up!

The healing is in the feeling.

~~~

13. If the pain doesn't clear up (for example, if it still has
weight), explore the feeling once more. Is there any
spot on the surface against which you're resisting,
fighting, trying to contain or control? (For example,
sometimes we're trying to subconsciously push the
pain out, rather than accept it.) If so, relax that
effort. Other times we may hold onto pain, believing
that it's protecting us from a deeper discomfort (e.g.,
loss). If so, ask the pain to be your ally in healing
that deeper discomfort. Let yourself continue feeling
the sensation of the pain, without resistance,
judgment, or expectation.

~ ~ ~

14. Stay with this sensual experience all the way from
the beginning, through the middle, past the end.
Listen. Keep breathing. Give thanks.

~ ~ ~

As you accept the power to heal, you'll find that an amazing
gift becomes available: the expanded ability to consciously receive
information from the unknown depths of your Being.

A few sources for deeper information you might not have
thought of:

The Physical Body: We often try to dominate it with vitamins
and exercise, prescriptions and surgery—in an effort to avoid pain
and even death. Could be, our bodies aren't prisons, but teachers.
Within each cell exists an innate intelligence that knows what's

needed for perfect balance. Could it be your body just wants you to listen?

Your Relationships with Others: Jesus said, "Love thy neighbor as thyself"—because your neighbor is your own Unknown Self, made visible. Could it be, we are such powerful beings that whenever we need to see more deeply, we open up to someone crossing our path who can demonstrate a given lesson?

Your Wants and Desires: As I'll explain in Chapter 11, your wants and desires are vital, powerful tools ready to help you access your fullest potential.

When Are the Next Messengers Due?

They'll show up at just the right time—whenever you're ready, even though you may not think so!

Pains, remember, are a valid part of reality, which is unfolding exactly as it should. The more you accept the subtler, quieter messengers and learn to heed them, the less you'll need to create anguish and discomfort for yourself.

Imbalances will always occur. (Even Olympic skaters take a tumble now and then.) So try as we might, you and I will never lose our ability to create more pain. If we did, we would also lose our freedom of choice, and become slaves.

Remember, your pains and mine are corrective devices, to keep us aimed at our Larger Target of . . . (*I know mine; you'll have to fill in this blank yourself; see Chapter 13!*). And as your aim grows ever more accurate, these pesky little messengers become smaller, ever smaller, and easier to heal.

Glossary
Translating Pain—What "Bad" Feelings Mean

As you accept emotional pain, you'll soon find that it's generated by similar patterns of lies or distorted thoughts. (I find that guilt, for example, tells me that I've stopped focusing on my sacredness, my oneness with God.) I suggest you explore these suggestions and definitions.

Abandonment: Mistaken belief that someone has shunned you. In reality, you've somehow abandoned your own sacredness.

Anger/resentment: Belief that denying your true wants and desires will make you happy. Belief that if you hide your fears, you'll be more accepted. Denial of your desires. Anger often hides the fear of feeling powerless. Often we get stuck in anger, believing we're really angry with others, when we're actually angry with ourselves! Blaming others for our pain often produces anger.

Anxiety: Mistaken notion that your choices and opportunities are limited, that the universe isn't unfolding as it should. Fear that opportunities are few and far between—and that when they do show up, you don't deserve them.

Betrayal: Hidden belief that you've sold out yourself and/or your relationship with God.

Boredom: Ongoing belief that the present moment isn't as it should be. Belief that there's no opportunity to contribute to the present. A subtle messenger indicating an area of growth that's asking to be accepted.

Defeat: Belief that failures undermine your validity. Mistaken notion that the present circumstance isn't supposed to be happening. Refusal to release an expectation.

Depression: Mistaken belief that denying feelings is a long-term solution to pain.

Despair: Mistaken notion that you've lost the ability to choose. The idea that the current situation is lacking in healing options. Belief that not having expressed your potential causes separation from God and from your own sacredness.

Disappointment: Erroneous expectation that what *should* be is more important than what *is*. Sometimes, the mistaken notion that God is telling you that you're undeserving.

Emptiness/Nothingness: Mistaken belief that you're really nothing, unworthy of even being loved. Avoidance of accepting your unique sacredness.

Fear: Mistaken belief that you're really incapable, and separate from the unlimited power around us. A manifestation of beliefs in limitation.

Fear of being different: Mistaken idea that others (and not you) are the source of your being accepted, validated, and approved of.

Fear of chaos: Unwillingness to experience life in the present. The mistaken belief you're in control of life. Explore also the fears of losing your power to heal and losing the power to love yourself.

Fear of failure: Belief that your mistakes have invalidated you.

Fear of impotence: "But I can't!" Mistaken belief that the universe doesn't love you, that whatever support you need isn't available right now. Mistrust of the universe, mistrust of life.

Fear of not being loved: Failure to notice that you've stopped loving yourself.

Fear of ridicule: Mistaken belief that you aren't valid when others judge you or seek to diminish you. Belief that failure invalidates the self.

Fear of the unknown: Belief that the universe is unloving, if not hostile.

Feeling lost: Thinking that because you cannot see options or choices, you have none. Also, belief in the adversarial nature of the universe; not allowing the universe to love you.

Feeling overwhelmed: Belief that you're not able to deal with challenges. Defining yourself as a failure, due to judgement of circumstances.

Grieving: Erroneous notion that death and loss are inevitable. Most of us started bemoaning loss the moment we learned of death, not even considering that life is inevitable. Accepting ownership of our death-related fears helps nurture more life, and "living each day to its fullest." Whenever we choose to die, we can do so in a way that expands our ability to love. Maybe we're not the victims, but the initiators, of our physical demise.

Guilt: Believing you're unworthy and deserve punishment, because of mistakes, failures, "bad" desires and choices. Belief that any lesson could be unforgivable; that whatever lesson you're learning is the wrong one.

Humiliation: Mistaken belief that your validity is based on not making mistakes. "This failure means I'm a loser."

Impatience: Fervent belief that if you accept the present, you'll invalidate yourself. Adopting an attitude of pain-avoidance, selecting a future scenario as an antidote, and trying to control the present accordingly.

Loneliness: Misconception that you're separate from the Oneness of All That Is.

Mistrust: Notion that you should protect yourself from pain, rather than heal it. Unwillingness to see yourself as the cause of your own experience.

Need or desire to control: Mistaken thought that you lack the power to heal pain, but must manage and avoid it instead. A necessary component is blaming others for your own pain.

Neediness: Mistaken belief that someone else can do a better job of loving or healing you than you can. Denial in expressing your true desires.

Powerlessness: Longstanding belief that you're incapable. Notion that experience will cause you to lose your identity. Resistance to being honest about wants and desires.

Procrastination: Belief that you're incapable of facing your own goals; fear of failing in your purpose.

Rejection: Notion that your negative thoughts are really true; belief that others really do have power to validate or invalidate you.

Repugnance: Deeply held, erroneous notion that a lesson or condition isn't here to expand the growth and expression of your unlimited self.

Sadness: Mistaken belief that because someone or something is no longer present, you can no longer experience your connection with that person or thing.

Self-loathing: Denying and invalidating your experiences and emotions. Questioning your innocence. Belief in undeservingness and diminishment.

Separation: Mistaken notion that your perception of yourself as isolated is accurate. Denial of the fundamental Oneness of All That Is.

Shame: Mistaken notion that God withholds love from you for your failures, mistakes and sins. Belief that a condition can sever your loving relationship with God. Deep invalidation of self. Mistaken belief that condemnation and punishment rectify shortcomings.

Struggle: Behavior reflecting an attempt to control shame, rather than heal it.

Sympathy: Emotional reaction to the belief that another is weaker than their pain. Not to be confused with compassion and empathy.

Unworthiness: Mistaken belief that your judgments/ diminishments of yourself and others are valid.

CHAPTER SEVEN
From Stagnation to Growth: Dancing with Energy

While exploring these experiments and definitions, take it for granted that there are many unseen, hidden energies waiting to serve you. To access them, first you must acknowledge that they *might* exist!

On a most practical level, every one of us enjoys a unique relationship with the energy of the universe—that powerful stuff that fuels the Milky Way and the Pleiades and our own local star. It surrounds and supports all life on earth (and who knows where else?), and empowers the act of creation. Reality is a vast invisible network of unending energy streams, flowing to destinations that will become physical and visible at some future moment. I suggest, further, that each of us is a unique vibration of this energy, able to focus our awareness so that the energy around us—of which we are a part! —responds.

Ignore the energy surrounding this physical existence, and you ignore a very powerful, loving, and responsive ally. If I acknowledge nothing more than the reality that I can see, touch, and measure, I'll find life a struggle. Circumstances seem to overpower my experience; my choices seem to have little impact.

Often clients ask me, "How can I become aware of energy?" And my answer is, "You already are!" Subconsciously, we're all responding to one another's energies. Sit quietly with your eyes closed, and you can probably feel when someone silently walks into the room.

Some of my clients can see energy around others, in the form of the aura. Others feel it, still others merely suspect its presence, but all of us can see its effects. The reality we're living in is the physical materialization of our collective energies. (I haven't noticed any major gaps in reality lately, so I presume that energy is always manifesting; that our thoughts are always creating. Does this seem overwhelming to you? People who've had their sight restored, never having known vision before, report a sense of being similarly overwhelmed, because they never expected to find something everywhere they look.)

I'm suggesting that by using conscious choice, you and I can expand our awareness of energy and, in so doing, more readily access our individual and collective potentials.

Could it be that the energy of this universe is equally aware of you and awaiting your command? Once you accept this unique relationship, you can then tackle the job of communicating with this energy, so that it fully serves you and the contributions you seek to create. Conscious use of energy means training your mind to serve your highest good.

Serge King, a Huna Kahuna, speaks of effectiveness as a measure of truth. In other words, the effectiveness of your ability to create depends on your conscious access to your truth.

A simple example will illustrate this: Next time you're planning a trip of at least 20 miles, imagine all the trials and tribulations you can. Consider yourself deeply put out by this excursion—and then notice the experience (and success) of the first leg of your journey. Then, on your return, reverse your focus: Think of the journey as a delight. See yourself enjoying the trip, and imagine other travelers pleased to cross your path. Again, note the quality of your experience.

I'm going to assume that you'd vastly prefer a happy journey. And the effectiveness of that manifestation depends on whether we focus on the truth of who we are and our truly joyful opportunities to be together. Remember, the more you accept your present experience (and conversely, the less you resist what you *don't* like), the better able you'll be to manifest what you truly want.

For a working definition, let's call energy the medium that transports thought into manifestation. Energy allows both your hopes and fears to become reality (at least until you start to doubt the idea—so if you believe that your thoughts don't matter, then they'll be much less effective!).

Do your imaginings support this relationship, or hinder it?

So, before expanding our study of energy, we must explore any beliefs that will impede its effectiveness.

Mistaken Notions About the Use of Energy

1) *The Universe doesn't respond to my thoughts. The Universe is an unconscious, inanimate place, with no recognition of my unique being.* Many people actually believe the Universe is hostile! They're startled to hear that if they hold the Universe as an enemy, it *manifests* as an enemy—and, conversely, that if they see the Universe as loving, it manifests accordingly.

Experiment with this idea! Put it to the test! On even-numbered days, imagine the world as your enemy. On odd-numbered days, make the universe your ally. You may be surprised to find how closely the universe lives up—and down—to your expectations.

(Listen closely: You might just hear God giggling!)

~ ~ ~

2) *My spoken—and unspoken—words have no power. What we think and say has no effect on the reality unfolding around us.* This distortion stems from the insecurities expressed in that age-old question to God, "What is man, that Thou should'st be mindful of him?"

Too many people believe they're insignificant, that they make no difference. Truth is, we're so powerful that if we start to imagine ourselves as insignificant, that's how we appear to ourselves. We imagine a distortion or a limitation, and presto! —it manifests. But just because we can imagine the self as diminished, that doesn't diminish the self—it just appears so. Sadly, too often, we believe the illusion! Collectively, our thoughts and desires make up the very fabric of our culture and environment around us.

3) *I need extensive training before any of this will work.* Do you think you need to be some kind of authority (or worse, possess sufficient credentials) before energy will respond to your directions and desires? Who you are is enough!

4) *If I make a mistake using energy, I'll lose the chance to go further in my lessons.* You'll find that in this physical domain, energy seems to be a loving teacher who sends gentle reminders when we're in error. Whenever we ignore these messengers, they simply get louder. Thus we learn to listen.

At times, as you and I gain greater power to create consciously, we may try to flaunt that skill for our own aggrandizement. But you'll find that trying to boost your ego and dramatize your importance will gradually diminish your access to energy.

5) *I can use energy to help me control others.* I invite you to experiment with this mistaken notion! You'll find, I suspect, that ultimately, any attempts you make to dominate others will simply distance you from your own power. If you're seeking revenge or

preparing to go into battle, chances are you're not going to be aware of the subtle communications necessary to use energy effectively.

Keep in mind that energy follows your thoughts. Focus on limitations, consciously or subconsciously, and you contribute to the stagnation of energy.

The trick is to notice when energy is flowing and when it's not. Energy can get stuck in your mind, your emotions, your body and your environment. Stagnant energy produces pain and imbalance. It manifests as unresolved conflict, upsets, and separation in our relationships with ourselves and others. It's not available to serve manifestation, thus creating the condition we call being "stuck" in life. Too many of us have become so accustomed to being stuck that we don't expect life to be any different. The rare experiences of growth seem to be miracles, rather than the true nature of life— the way existence is designed to be.

Getting stuck takes a certain exertion. After all, energy wants to move! To retard its flow, you must maintain focus (often subconsciously) on a limitation or distortion. As you become aware that your limiting thoughts produce pain, you can learn to think so that reality reflects the natural progression of growth in your life.

Experiment #19

Acceptance / Resistance

This is an easy one.

1. Simply resist whatever's occurring in your life today, and notice your discomfort.

2. Tomorrow, accept all of your day's events as they transpire, and notice the sensations associated with growth and progression.

To see the results of your relationship with energy—and see where you're focusing it—simply observe the flow of life around you. Be conscious of your present reality and the quality of your thoughts. Energy is always manifesting in—and *as*—this present reality. Whatever each of us needs for growth is always present. Stagnant areas of life carry a very simple message: Whatever limitations you're focusing on need to be cleansed, or cleared away.

John walked into my office one day, complaining that he felt stuck in his life. Feeling isolated and unloved, he'd been failing at one relationship after another for the past ten years. As a boy, he'd tried to dominate his younger sister while rebelling against his mother's control. Still feeling guilty about this period of his life, John feared that he'd never be able to love his family again. He was understandably reluctant to focus on the pain associated with these past events, but ultimately, he relented.

"John," I asked, "what do you think it would take for you to be free of your past?"

"I'd have to know that God has forgiven me," he replied.

"But what if God has already forgiven you?"

He paused for a moment. "Then I guess I would have to forgive myself."

I could tell that this was a revelation for him. "What would it take," I continued, "for you to love the part of yourself that went through these experiences? What would it take for you to look back at those times as a valuable lesson that helped you grow?"

"I can see that I'd have to accept that part of my life," John said.

"Can you see how all of those experiences taught you something about how you truly feel about your family?"

"Yes," he said. "It's obvious that I really love them, and that I want them to know it."

Over the next several weeks, he had a number of deep conversations with his sister and mother. For the first time in his life, he was able to apologize for his childhood behavior. John found his family not only forgiving, but delighted that he was able to open his heart to them. He, in turn, reclaimed a level of love for himself that he'd abandoned years before.

Many of us treat our lessons and our growth the way John did. We condemn ourselves, rather than learning to love ourselves in the midst of our learning. Perhaps "the still, small voice of God within" ultimately teaches us to love ourselves more fully. In mastering the art of learning, can we discover our own unique ways of doing so? Can we make it okay to learn, rather than believe that lessons mean that we still have a long way to go?

All too often we argue for the heavy-duty kneepads in life, because as kids, we fell when we tried to walk. Certainly the effective use of energy requires that you and I accept ourselves as complete—and still growing.

This universe we've created collectively has a strong healing vibration. When working on healing, big or small, try reconnecting yourself with the physical world. Take a walk outside in the fresh air, or a dip in the local lake or river. *Nature absorbs emotion.* Breathe deeply, and let your mind be open to any message your pain has to deliver. Take great joy in this experiment!

Effective use of energy requires that you be at peace with your body. That means accepting your ability to heal pain! (*See box.*)

Experiment #21

Imagining Energy

Use your awareness to become ever more conscious of energy. Perform this exercise whenever you become aware of any physical or emotional discomfort.

1. Where in your body does this sensation reside?

2. Sit quietly. Close your eyes. Breathe deeply. Focus your awareness on this painful location.

3. Imagine that the sensation has a specific shape.

4. Visualize a ball of white light, two to three inches in diameter, floating just inside the base of your skull, at the medulla oblongata.

5. Envision this sphere shooting a beam of white light directly to the physical location of your pain, completely enfolding the location.

6. Maintain this focus for at least 60 seconds, breathing deeply and evenly as you do.

~ ~ ~

7. Now, after one minute, how does your discomfort feel?

   Repeat this visualization as needed. Whenever your rational mind seeks to distract you, gently redirect the beam of white light from the top of your spine, over to *the area of pain.*

Energy follows thought, energy follows focus.

Please plant this idea deep within your grey cells.

What are so many ascended masters (like you and me!) doing here on earth? Mastering the use of energy, creating realities that faithfully reflect our greatest desires. Sure, we're already manifesting a common, collective reality. Yet the real work is about being able to create our own individual realities, consciously and compassionately, in concert with the collective One.

Communicating with Energy

We've explored how to heal pain by breathing through it, feeling it, and listening for its message. Now, I'd like to expand that further. I suggest that we can connect with the energy held within pain, and communicate with it. (Remember, energy follows thought!)

Many years ago, I found myself once again in a love affair with my teenage sweetheart, my first real love. After a few months, she suddenly ended it, and I suffered a heartfelt loss as my most cherished relationship ended—for the second time.

For weeks I moped around, racking my brain for some way to reverse the loss. I was obsessed with getting her back. I called, I wrote, I railed, I cried. I meditated daily, with little release. Anguished over my sorrow, I feared I had lost my last chance to ever love that deeply again.

Whenever I cling rabidly to a perspective, believing that point of view somehow protects my validity and deservingness, I usually must endure my pain for some time before I can hear its relevant message. And so, one afternoon, I finally received an insight: I had to examine what I really wanted.

I realized, after some introspection, that I wanted to experience my true validity for myself—and give up the need to be validated by a wonderful love affair. Further, fearing that I'd lost the great passion of my life, I wanted to expand my ability to love in the future.

All pain holds the key to healing—which in turn, brings an expansion of awareness. The next time I felt depressed about the loss of my love, I stilled myself and let myself feel deeply the loss and sadness. Then I consciously connected with the energy within the sadness: I simply imagined a receptive, willing essence within the sensation. Finally, I asked it to serve my intention to heal. I made that energy into an ally, asking it to help reclaim my ability to validate myself and my life once again.

At that very moment, I felt a wonderful release from pain. The whole experience expanded my ability to love.

Since then, I've found I can connect with the energy within any pain, and assign it a focused, specific purpose. The results have been truly magical, renewing my sense of life's wonder and majesty.

At the beginning, when you first start connecting with energy as a sensation, you need to deepen your awareness of it. Explore any emotional or physical sensation you encounter. Ask that the energy within the pain be available to your consciousness. This may occur as a feeling, a sensing, or perhaps a knowingness. Explore how the energy makes itself known to you, and trust your instincts. And keep practicing. Remember, your body, your Higher Self, and the universe all want you to learn this lesson!

Although we often define pain as nasty, energy is neither good nor bad. It's either moving or stagnant. Locked inside pain, energy is stagnant. By assigning that energy a purpose, you give it a new focus to get it moving again. And that's the whole point, the breakthrough: Stuck energy produces pain. Moving energy is creative, on its way to manifestation.

Experiment #23

The Energies Within Emotions

Can you ask the energies of . . .

Anger, to demonstrate your power to create?

Disappointment, to show you where recent developments can hasten your desires?

Fear, to let you face every challenge in a way that helps you grow?

Frustration and Impatience, to demonstrate that the universe is unfolding exactly as it should, easing the way for what you want to manifest?

Grief and Loss, to reclaim your passions and enthusiasms?

Guilt, to teach you your current lesson with greater ease, and even joy?

Loneliness, to expand your ability to love yourself and others?

Shame, to allow you to grasp your oneness with your God?

~ ~ ~

Experiment with these ideas, and create your own prayers for your own particular pains and desires.

Note the results!

To use energy effectively in *any* way, you must be clear and honest about what you truly desire. While there are no "bad" desires, it's certainly possible to pursue a want that produces pain. Do I want a new girlfriend to distract me from that previous grieving? To groom my ego's ruffled feathers? If so, this technique won't work!

Remember, resisting grief only produces more grief! If I look deeper into my desires, my true goals seem to be: 1) to heal the grief, and 2) to expand my experience of loving. But if I only want to avoid a previous loss, then I'll get a new relationship that lets me heal the loss. Period! That's all, folks! And I'll keep creating breakups until I heal from the original one.

Remember, the universe *always* manifests *whatever* you focus your awareness on—even if it's resistance. Any lesson that repeats itself is merely the universe telling you there's something that you're resisting.

To some observers, this is a *BIG* giggle, especially when it spans lifetimes!

~ ~ ~

We need to get beyond wanting simply to feel comfortable, happy, secure, or loved. Assuming we have the power to fulfill those goals on our own, seeking any outside something—or someone— to fulfill them is counterproductive! Whenever I make this kind of mistake, the universe always manifests some experience to remind me of my power to claim my power.

I've also found I can use the energy I used to squander on worrying about the future.

For example, when I began solstice meditations for my clients, the first one was scheduled for very early in the morning; and I worried that I might oversleep and miss it. The evening before, as I was planning to watch a movie, I caught myself fretting about oversleeping yet again. I decided to gather up all the energy packed within the worry and dedicate it—to restful sleep, an early awakening, and a beautiful outcome. Even though I was still a little apprehensive by the time I went to bed, I woke up early, feeling refreshed, and led a group meditation that was warmly received!

Personally, I find this use of Worry Energy definitely supports a favorable outcome of future events. First, locate the feeling of anxiety in your body. Then breathe, feel, listen, and then ask the energy for what you truly want.

Energy for New Beginnings

According to esoteric tradition, projects started at the new moon have a powerful opportunity for success. (Prison breaks should all be scheduled for the new moon!) Try an experiment by beginning projects at the new moon, or on the day of the summer or winter solstice.

Experiment #25

Assisted Beginnings

The Golden Mean is a mathematical concept, represented by the number 1.618033988749895 . . . (Let's call it 1.618, for short!) This ratio expresses perfect design throughout nature—as seen in the whorled seeds of a sunflower, the shell of the chambered nautilus, and the helix of DNA. Beginning a new creation? Write the first four digits of the Golden Mean at the head of your planning documents. See if this imbues the project with energy for reaching its ideal form, its greatest potential!

The abundance of this universe is often overlooked because we've forgotten our power to consciously direct energy to shape reality. This energy abounds, looking for conscious choice and commitment to direct it, as you learned in Chapter 4. The Hindus call it *prana* and long ago developed breathing practices to access this energy. Reiki healing is based on the notion that there exists an abundance of energy available for our healing in this moment. While we can imagine "energy shortages," in truth there is never any scarcity of energy when seeking a purpose.

Chapter Eight

The Hiding Self, The Emerging Self

L ife is simple—or should be. But to satisfy our craving to understand, we create structures and mental templates that feel secure. It's like picking up an old, familiar coat: "Yep, worn this jacket through 37 winters. Ain't died in it yet!" Trouble is, we get our legs stuck in the armholes of life, trying to force it to fit our expectations of how things should turn out. Expectations always are tailored too short!

In the Book of Genesis, God warned Adam and Eve not to eat the fruit of the tree of knowledge of good and evil. He knew that whenever humans try to be good and avoid being bad, they end up experiencing themselves as unworthy, unlovable, and undeserving.

You and I have spent lots of energy developing images—mental constructions—of ourselves. Most of my decisions were based on how I thought I *should* be, to elicit society's acceptance and approval. If other people felt good about me, didn't that prove I'm loveable?

I figured I should be smart, successful, and happy. I noticed, however, that I often experienced feelings of failure and stupidity, clumsiness and unworthiness. These feelings seemed to prove that I wasn't who I was supposed to be—so I hid these feelings from myself and devoted even more energy into developing a persona who was smart, successful, happy—and loved. Trouble is, these constructed self-images can vastly impede our energy and true power. When my clients don't consistently live out—or live up to—their "good" image, they punish themselves. They hide behind these images, use them to justify their dishonesties and try to control others' reactions—as in "You shouldn't behave that way around me! I'm too (*fill in the blank, but it better be good!*)."

Speaking personally, my "Good" image forced me to hide many of my most honest and true experiences, with statements like, "No, I'm *not* afraid," to "It's not cool to let you see how excited I am." I crafted that image to protect myself from my worst fears: that I truly might be a failure, and a loser, and a sinner—irrevocably tainted! Even after I quit writing ad copy, my mind kept right on doing so. Accordingly, most of my waking moments were spent trying to hide my "bad" facets, and proving they didn't exist.

~ ~ ~

As a child, I found my father very loving and supportive. Yet there were times of conflict when I feared him and judged myself a coward for not standing up to him. During one of my visits, after I was well into adulthood, my father and I got into an argument about how to treat Freckles, one of his hunting dogs. I had gone out back to play with Freckles, when my father shouted out the window, in a tone I heard as commanding and condescending at the same time.

I took a deep breath and shouted back, "I don't want to be controlled by you any longer!" We both got upset, and I walked out of his house, needing some time to myself. I'd finally voiced what I'd been afraid to say for so many years—yet surprisingly, I still felt ashamed of myself for being a coward.

Later, after he and I talked further, I realized he hadn't been trying to take away my choices about handling dogs, but only wanted to inform me about one of Freckles' idiosyncrasies. I was glad to come to peace about the argument, but still hadn't resolved my relationship with Ned the Coward.

Only several years later did it occur to me that I hadn't loved the aspect of myself that I'd condemned as cowardly. Rather than permit acceptance and healing, I'd been trying to control that aspect of myself. Once I understood that feeling fear doesn't mean cowardice, there came a wonderful release. I found greater strength to heal my fears, rather than needing to run from them.

Journal Exploration #27

Exploring the Image Disguise

Revealing these mental images leads you to a greater self-acceptance and, thus, expands your access to energy. In your journal or lined notebook, take as much space (or as little) as you need to complete the following:

1. On a left-hand page, complete these sentences:
    "My image of myself is . . ." *and*
    "I really think of myself as . . ."

2. On the facing, right-hand page, complete these sentences:
    "Other people's image of me is . . ." *and*
    "I want them to think of me as . . ."

3. Share the results of this exercise with three people.

Revealing these mental images to each other is a singularly empowering experience. It'll lead you to a greater self-acceptance, from whence arises all your real power.

~ ~ ~

In today's world, failure is the devil. We're far quicker to identify ourselves (and others) as failures than to view ourselves as sacred, divine beings. As a result, most of us carry a degraded self-image. We've forgotten that buying into self-diminishment condemns us to believe that others' opinions of us establish our validity. We label each other "losers," "stupid," "bad," "sick," "inadequate," "unlovable," "unworthy," and "wrong." We close our hearts, withhold love, justify isolation, seek revenge, and create beliefs that let us dehumanize each other. And we punish ourselves for our mistakes because we think that erases shame—the pain which is a natural result of invalidating the self. We honestly believe that mistakes tarnish our sacredness.

~ ~ ~

The soul is hardwired to keep itself safe and inviolate, under all circumstances. But if you believe you deserve punishment, that's what will manifest.

Funny thing, this attachment to punishment—as though if we get punished enough, we'll stop making mistakes. But again, if punishment truly nurtured growth, we'd be electing terrorists to public office. In fact, punishment seems to retard growth. Remember, resistance causes persistence; and punishment is the greatest expression of resistance. Visit a classroom where the teacher consistently diminishes errant pupils, and you'll find stuck children on their way to becoming stuck adults. Those teachers who encourage learning from mistakes have students who grow and take joy in expressing their unique talents.

Unconsciously, we create struggle in our lives as a convenient way to justify and deny failures. Many of us resist our own growth, struggling with our lessons rather than learning how to make them fun. We alone have the power to have fun while we learn — lessons aren't inherently fun or a struggle; rather, those qualities result from our own choices. We try to control our shame, rather than accept it as a signal of our deeper intent to discover our Unknown Self (*see Chapter 10*). And we sit around hoping for the day when we make our last mistake, so our punishment can finally end.

Remember, the feeling of shame is a great messenger, but as a belief, it's useless. Many of us excel at procrastination, because it helps us avoid being seen as failures. But guess what? You'll never be finished making mistakes—they're too valuable! Our mistakes are actually lessons, truly the footsteps that lead to the joyful expression of our full potential.

Experiment #29

Using the Hidden Energy in Punishment

Perform this exercise when you are judging yourself as a failure, or a disappointment.

1. Locate any painful feelings in your body. Breathe as you accept them.

    ~ ~ ~

2. Complete the Heal-A-Hurt Exercise on page 72.

3. Ask your body to help you experience clearly what you truly desire during this experience of punishment. (That is, do you want to heal the pain of unworthiness? Experience a greater expression of love? Forgive yourself?)

4. Ask your body to help you in manifesting what you truly want.

5. Give thanks.

Mired in revenge and punishment? Ask the tremendous energy invested in those goals to nourish your ability to forgive! Validating aspects of yourself that you most dislike is a major challenge. But as you learn to validate (and heal) these parts of yourself, you can begin to appreciate others whom you've judged and condemned.

Have you considered telling the universe that you've been punished enough? Of course, most of us think we have evidence to the contrary, but I'd like to suggest you've created all the evidence anyway. See if it nurtures you to give up the need to be punished for one week.

Pull out all the stops! Give up punishment forever! The universe can count on you to grow without bring chastised. Are you willing to trust yourself this way? As an innocent child of the divine universe, you can learn lessons however you choose. Yes, choices have consequences. But by banishing punishment, consequences become tools for learning and validation.

When you give up attachments to punishment, you access new energies for learning, growth and love. You automatically lose the need to defend your self-image and move toward being at peace with your "complete" self.

Experiment #31

Creating an End to Punishment

1. Sit quietly and imagine yourself at some point in your future, when you and God have decreed that you have been punished enough. This doesn't mean you'll never make another mistake, simply that you can be trusted to grow and learn without being beaten into it.

    ~ ~ ~

    Allow yourself to fully experience whatever feelings occur.

2. Accept this decree, and imagine how you would love to celebrate the event. Who would you like to invite? Where would this event take place? What would you wear?

3. What provisions would you make to remind yourself of this decree, should you fall back into the habit of punishing yourself? (Breathing helps.)

    ~ ~ ~

4. Upon accepting this decree, would you be willing to give up the need to punish others, as well?

5. Declare general amnesty. (Why wait another minute?) Breathe and give thanks.

Growth isn't going to stop. Change is the ongoing process of life, and I suspect God also continues to grow. That means we'll constantly be facing the unknown—and our choices, inevitably, will sometimes produce mistakes. Stop resisting them—all of them! —and you get to experience mistakes for the"blessons" they really are.

~ ~ ~

One of the most unfortunate blind spots in our society is that we don't realize that our thoughts about ourselves comprise our own self-image—a persona, if you will, that masks our true self. Yet whenever we buy into beliefs of unworthiness and undeservingness, often we create a false image that I call the"Bad" Self. Others privately call it the Failure Self, the Loser Self, or the Unlovable Self. Like most of us, however, I try to prove that the "Bad" Ned doesn't exist.

Just like my clients, my "Bad" Self wants to be heard and accepted—not indulged or ignored. It helps me learn the worth of all of my aspects. By exploring whatever pain my"Bad" Self holds, I've found a deep reservoir of energy to love and desire to contribute that my own self-judgment had obscured. Having established communication with my "Bad" Self, I can ask it to support healing—its greatest desire. Without communicating with and healing your"Bad" Self, you can't access all the dimensions of your unlimited Self. Access to your own power and energy is vastly compromised.

Journal Exploration #33

Embracing Your "Bad" Self

1. List the broken commitments, failed relationships, people from whom you've withheld your love.

2. List the self-judgments you hold about the list in question # 1.

3. In terms of your relationships with others, what would it cost if you had to stop judging, invalidating yourself, and promoting your "Bad" Self? For example, would your friends resent you, if you stopped saying you can't face your addiction to chocolate?

4. Close your eyes and breathe. Imagine your "Bad" Self sitting across from you, feeling a great desire to communicate with you. What's needed to start the dialogue with your "Bad" Self?

~ ~ ~

5. What pains do you ask your "Bad" Self to hide?

6. What does your "Bad" Self truly want? What healing is it seeking? How would it love to express itself?

7. Ask your "Bad" Self for support in *fully* forgiving yourself. Ask it to fully support you in accepting your unique validity. Teach the "Bad" Self to breathe!

~ ~ ~

Journal Exploration #35

Viewing Failure as an Ally

Answer these questions:

1. How have your failures and mistakes contributed to your life? (As a toddler, falling down certainly helped you master walking!) Focus especially on the big mistakes, the ones you have yet to forgive.

2. How would you *like* to use the energy contained within your mistakes and failures? (For example, can you ask the energy involved in withholding love to further your expressions of loving?)

3. Should you ever repeat the same mistake, would you be willing to love yourself in that moment, and support your intention to master the lesson? Would you be willing to share this lesson with others who cross your path?

~ ~ ~

Ever watch anyone trying to prove his self-worth—something undeniable and inherent within each of us? What a waste of time! Our definitions of ourselves, usually based on judgmental dichotomies of good/bad, right/wrong, beautiful/ugly, lead us to conclude that we're not worthy. We're trained to deal with this experience by controlling it.

Reward is one of the great controlling tools we use to prove that we're worthy (rather than simply accepting our own worth). Whenever we personally claim the truth of our eternal value, we begin to see the power that each of us has—the power to hold ourselves above violation. Yet, all too often, to "remind" ourselves of our value, we hand ourselves rewards. Some religions even teach that good means God is rewarding us, while pain is His punishment.

One afternoon, I was working with Shelly, a single mom who was weaning herself off drugs. She had done considerable work on forgiving her failings, yet she acknowledged a subconscious urge toward self-destruction.

"Shelly," I asked, having just been hit with a flash of insight, "if you stopped punishing yourself, is there something else you'd have to give up?"

I watched as she considered the question. Clearly, it had meaning for her, and she gave herself a moment to explore her inner awareness. Suddenly, her face brightened, and she said, "I see it! If I had to stop beating myself up, it would cost me the rewards I allow myself!"

Shelly had discovered how entangled punishments and rewards really are—because they both depend on the idea that our validity can be compromised, and must be proven. As she explored the reflections of this belief in her life, Shelly was able to relax her dependence on drugs and shift her focus toward accepting and loving herself.

Journal Exploration #37

The Pain Hidden in Rewards

1. Over a week's time, keep a journal record of all the rewards you give yourself. Refrain from any judging. Simply note the rewards, and when you bestowed them.

2. Notice any patterns. How consistently do your rewards compensate for a painful experience? For example, do you always give yourself ice cream after an argument with your spouse, partner, or close friend?

3. As you notice patterns emerging, in a quiet meditation, ask yourself, "Where in this behavior do I believe or feel I'm undeserving, powerless or unworthy?" Write down the answers.

4. Explore the painful feelings among these patterns. Use whatever healing exercise is effective for you. Beneath the pain hidden by reward look for messages that speak of greater desires to express your talents.

5. Give thanks.

Giving up rewards doesn't mean you can't pursue your desires. It just means you'll stop seeking rewards to make yourself feel better. If you're capable of healing pain, why distract yourself with a gold medal? Replace the need to reward yourself with something even better—your power to heal and thus, manifest. Ask the universe for whatever you want, and honor yourself by accepting what shows up as exactly what's needed for your dreams to come true.

It'll take me this whole book to explain how simple this is! The power to create becomes available only when we've accepted that we're deserving, that we're one with our God, and have every right to be the unique expression of God that we really are.

Can you accept the challenge of deserving? Can you give up the need to prove it, and simply accept it? Can you stop asking life to validate your deservingness, and do this vital job for yourself? Experiment with this challenge with gusto, breathing as you go!

~ ~ ~

Remember, every pain indicates that you've withheld energy in some way. And whenever you've withheld energy from someone else, you also withhold from yourself, on the same pretext. (If I can't love myself because I'm dishonest, I'll condemn you for your dishonesty.)

I vividly remember making real progress toward giving up my need to diminish myself. Thinking I'd finished working on that lesson, one day I found myself condemning a friend who was struggling with the same problem—he was judging himself for having failed in his job. I was very surprised to find myself judging him for a lesson I thought I'd just mastered!

At that time, I didn't realize my judgment that it was "bad" to stay stuck in a lesson. Once I did learn to forgive myself on that point, I automatically felt greater compassion for others fighting the same hassle. This helped me support clients who were stuck in their own lessons, rather than impede their growth.

So that I might learn a little more compassion, was the universe sending me people still working on lessons I'd just completed?

Could it be, other people's mistakes are challenges for us to examine our own errors? Whenever you start comparing yourself to others, mistrust your conclusions!

Since then, I've kept training myself to clean up judgments of others. Whenever I catch a judgment in my mind, I change my thinking and actively extend myself to help that person. Recently, after mentally blaming a neighbor for not maintaining his car, I offered to help repair it. In doing so, I opened up a more honest and friendly relationship, replacing distance and mistrust.

~ ~ ~

Hidden Energies in the Past

Cleaning up the past, I've discovered, helps us experience richer, more powerful energy in the present.

When I was much younger, during a road trip through the Southwest, I snuck a friend into a motel room for the evening without paying. Years later, I wrote a letter to that motel: "Would you let me know the additional charges for an additional guest in that room?"

Their response overwhelmed me. "Thanks for your letter, and your intent to correct the oversight. We don't want to accept any payment, but do invite you to stay with us whenever you are in the area."

One of the best ways to express love for yourself is to clean up any messes you've created, so that you needn't lug unfinished business through your daily life. Few actions can free up more creative energy. Few actions so powerfully align us with our path of growth.

From my many lessons in doing this, I've learned that step one is to stop blaming anyone else for pain you suffered in the situation.

Otherwise, you can't claim ownership of your own past baggage. If any event still holds pain for you, there's something you need to clean up—if only in your relationship with yourself.

Yet when I address this energy-building idea of cleaning up the past, people often complain that the job's too big. *Completing the past doesn't take forever.* It may take only a moment. Sometimes all that's needed is simply giving up the belief that pain is a requirement to clean up our mistakes. Completing the past does take dropping self-judgment, plus a willingness to step into the unknown! And while the unknown may include others' reactions after you've opened up the past for completion, you can trust that at our core, none of us wants to be dragging around more excess baggage.

~ ~ ~

CHAPTER NINE
Acknowledging Your Greatness

M any years ago, during my seminar-leader training with
est, I was delivering a presentation to a group of fellow
students. I was feeling uncomfortable in my attempts to relax and
speak in front of the group when Paul, one of the trainers, suddenly
walked up from the back of the room and interrupted me: "Hey,
Ned! Are you a weird kid trying to play it straight?"

I was stunned. But his question prompted me to explore how
I'd rejected my own uniqueness. For most of my life, I'd felt
"different" and had tried to hide it, so that I'd be accepted. Paul's
question let me stop asking others to accept me as a way of proving
I'm okay—and instead let me start validating myself just as I am.

Greatness isn't relegated to only a few, although myths and
beliefs suggest otherwise. In *Twelfth Night* (Act Two, Scene V),
Shakespeare wrote, "Some are born great, some achieve greatness,
and some have greatness thrust upon 'em."

That familiar passage is directly preceded by an
admonition—which is very seldom quoted: ". . . Be not afraid
of greatness . . ."

But many of us are! Sadly, too few of us dare accept our true
potential.

"He's good looking—and he knows it!"

"She's so stuck up!"

"He's awfully proud of himself!"

Bragging about your gifts in public is a major taboo. We often
understate our talents so that others won't accuse us of harboring

an inflated picture of ourselves. But this behavior often keeps us from acknowledging our gifts—thus limiting the contribution we can make to the world.

Experiment #39

Revealing Resistance to Your Potential

1. Everyday, for seven days, spend a few moments quieting your mind, breathing ~ ~ ~ and sitting in a relaxed state. Connect with your own inner sense of being. Ask your subconscious to reveal all the hidden blocks that keep you from accepting your full potential.

2. During these seven days, spend some time observing what shows up in your personal reality. Allow yourself full access to your feelings, even when they make no sense. Breathe!

~ ~ ~

3. Watch for messages that point to your hidden resistance to accepting your greatness. Give thanks!

We're taught to define greatness with external criteria—not realizing that doing so diminishes the profound value of uniqueness, inherent within each of us. Using these external considerations, we can never truly measure our individual greatness.

Our rational minds are designed to validate any belief we program into it. And, as children, we develop the ability to justify anything! Yes, the most prominent celebrity might get the most visibility, but how can we measure the gifts of that tireless, enormously helpful grade-school teacher who doesn't get quoted on the front page? Consider how much the mother of the man who made your shoes has contributed to your life!

The more you deny your own unique beauty, the less you experience your profound connection with the world. This narrows your ability to perceive the loveliness all around you—a great shame, since we humans are hard-wired to respond to even the smallest touches of beauty. We often use the resultant pain to justify further isolation from the world, rather than heeding its message: to accept the inner beauty that has always been ours.

All too often we despair, thinking we'll lose our ability to perceive this greatness. Yet all of us want our lives to make a difference. We want to expand the beauty in this world, be creative, express our potentials, grow and heal! As you become more open to energy and healing, you'll naturally rediscover that life is beautiful everywhere. If anything, beauty is consistent. Deep within everything is that spark of the Divine that deeply inspires us all.

~ ~ ~

I believe that if we commit to accepting our individual greatness, it can initiate the next phase of our evolution as a species. Each of us is learning what it takes to be honest about our failures and successes, our winnings and losses, so that they do not prove or disprove our greatness.

Privately, I resoundingly encourage you to be honest about your talents, gifts, and potentials—even when others disagree. I'm not suggesting that you seek to compare your greatness with others, and thus justify diminishing anyone else. Rather, I'd encourage that your recognition of your own greatness support you in a greater ability to perceive greatness in others.

~ ~ ~

A helpful hint from your Aunt Eloise: Accepting your own individual greatness lets you access greater energy! I'm not telling you to become conceited, but acknowledging your gifts and talents creates many more opportunities to express energy in your own unique way.

Journal Exploration #41

Investigating Greatness

1. List five excuses you use to hide your talents, gifts, and potentials from others—and yourself. Put another way, list the ways you resist your own potential.

2. When did you sell out your integrity, and not forgive yourself?

3. To whom do you need to apologize for not pursuing your potential? Who needs to apologize to you for not pursuing theirs?

4. What failures have you accused yourself of, and not forgiven?

5. When have you closed your heart to others and blamed them for that choice?

6. When you sell out your greatness, what does it cost you?

7. When you sell out your greatness, what does it cost others?

~ ~ ~

Too many of us spend our lives punishing, diminishing, and withholding love from ourselves. You and I must learn how to give up judging ourselves, before we can stop imprisoning ourselves by our limitations. We're meant to commit to our own validity, so that even our worst pain and greatest failings can't diminish our own sacredness.

I suspect you and I undertook this life-journey to discover our larger dimensions. That entails seeking out the sacredness of every individual—and each individual experience. You and I don't need a "test" or crisis to prove ourselves. As the offspring of an infinite, loving universe, we're more valuable than our rational minds can ever possibly grasp!

Recently, my stockbroker called to inform me that a bond issue I'd invested in had dropped 70% in value!

My emotions sank. My expectations and beliefs about being a success had been violated. As a successful investor, I was supposed to be *making* enough money to at least pay taxes on my gains. I felt taken advantage of, conned and duped.

Hanging up the phone, I blamed my broker, his research department, and the management of the company that issued the bond. Finally, I stopped my mind chatter long enough to breathe. When I accepted the discomfort and asked for its message, I realized the pain was indicating how I'd given away my validity to yet another outside source. Since the bond had gone down in value, so had I—and obviously, the company was to blame for my invalidation.

This experience forced me to explore how much I'd identified with my financial success. I was challenged to see how that was costing me my ability to heal and affirm love—even for myself.

(When I exercise my stubborn muscle, lessons like this usually demand some high tuition payments!)

Our innate worth, our sovereignty can never be diminished, so where's the need to prove it? If you're *truly* unique (that bears repeating!), who's the ultimate authority? You, and you alone! God Him/Herself could show up on your doorstep, singing the praises of your uniqueness. But if you couldn't accept your greatness, it couldn't possibly manifest in your life. You're the CEO at the job of validating yourself! No circumstance, no outside authority, no mistake is powerful enough to invalidate your worth. When you can trust yourself to validate yourself, regardless of success or failure, you will tap into a level of energy that profoundly helps you express your potentials.

We're halfway through this book. Time to make sure that your rational mind isn't working against you. *High* time you gave up the need to prove your validity!

First off, stop comparing your talents—and your experiences— with anyone else's. Whenever you compare, sooner or later you wind up concluding, "I am less than . . ." Comparisons set up a menu for self-judgment. And whenever you denigrate or resist any aspect of yourself, your access to energy is greatly diminished.

Doubting your own talents is a convenient way to avoid facing the responsibility of using them. But even after you agree to heal this fear, you'll still retain the power to doubt yourself. One day, an angel might show up on your doorstep and declare that you are holy, sacred, and perfect. Even when that day arrives, however, you'll still have an outer mind able to doubt yourself. Even when we've evolved to the point of walking on water, I think we'll still be able to doubt, asking, "Why can't we be levitating?"

Why not focus the energy you've invested in doubt in a different direction: namely, toward a growing acceptance of your unlimited self? Struggle or sacredness, it's always your choice—and what joy to discover you and I are not here to prove our greatness, simply to share it!

I used to suppress my unbridled enthusiasm because it seemed to make other people uncomfortable. All too many people told me, "Grow up, Ned!" It took some conscious effort to be honest about my joy and heal my embarrassment at being myself.

You and I are unique in our talents, gifts and potentials. And that's as it should be, since you and I are traveling on unique paths, creating and mastering unique lessons.

Experiment #43

Expressing Your Uniqueness

1. Find a quiet place, without distractions. Still your body and mind. If music helps you relax, turn it on.

2. Write yourself a letter, as though it came from a loving universe that's attentive, aware, and proud of your personal journey through eternity.

3. As you write, breathe. Let your entire life—your accomplishments, your lessons, successes and failures—be fully acknowledged. Let this acknowledgment in; be willing to receive it.

    Having difficulty writing the letter? Ask a person you trust—who knows you well—to write a few lines that honestly acknowledge you.

4. Accept what's written in this letter. Accept all feelings and sensations associated with this experience. Breathe!

    ~ ~ ~

    Ask the universe to help you accept your uniqueness.

    Give thanks.

    Give up any sense of obligation, or fear that this acknowledgment limits your choices. Re-read the letter every three days, until you experience the universe's love for you.

    Give thanks. Learn to love yourself as fully as do the sun, rain, air and earth.

Experiment #45

Using Your Sacredness

Anytime you find yourself in an unpleasant circumstance . . .

1. Quiet yourself and go within. Focus on a place inside where you accept, without question, your sacred uniqueness.

2. Welcome the unpleasant circumstance, event, or person into your consciousness.

3. Ask the event (or person), "Did you enter my life so as to support my greater growth?" If the answer is yes, then continue. If the answer is no, ask the person or event to pass on from you now. Remove it from your conscious focus.

   Continue on with your day, giving thanks for your greatness.

   ~ ~ ~

4. If the event or person is there for your greater growth, ask it to deliver any message it has that will support that growth. Sit quietly for a few minutes, listening. If you receive a message, consider how you can integrate it into your life. Give thanks and excuse the messenger. If you don't hear any message, trust that within the next three days, a fresh insight will appear to support your growth.

5. Note results. And again, permit the messenger to depart in peace!

When you accept your own sacredness, perhaps the greatest blessing is the knowledge that no matter what the circumstances, you have the power to hold yourself above violation and diminishment. Such love! Such power!

~ ~ ~

CHAPTER TEN
Your Multi-Dimensional Self

You and I are far more than we think we are, more than we can possibly conceive. I've watched hundreds of people safely walk across eight-hundred-degree coals. I've seen clients heal chronic, incurable conditions in a heartbeat and release decades-long debilitating emotions in a thrice. I've been blessed with countless flashes of knowingness that couldn't be accounted for through my education or experience. I've watched a multitude of us direct our thoughts in such a way that reality immediately reflects our intentions.

This all points to nothing if not to the fact that each of us is far more than an individualized human being, existing within the bounds of time and space. We are unlimited, eternal beings, each capable of bringing greater dimensions of the Self into the here and now.

~ ~ ~

We are both engaged, you and I, in a mighty, joyful struggle to reclaim our sacred, multi-dimensional selves. To remind us of this path, we'll do anything—including create great pain, if that's the only way we'll hear the message.

As you read this book, realize that you're more than your body, thoughts, possessions, personality or talents. Consider yourself as Divine—really! Think of yourself as an eternal presence, a unique expression of the Unlimited, with the power to create your own reality.

Otherwise, these ideas won't make sense to you. Otherwise,

you'll think that circumstances are more powerful than you are.

If you still believe that outside events are restricting your choices, then you might as well pass this book to someone else. But if you've had a taste of your own power and infinity, sleep with this book under your pillow—use it to support a greater awareness of your unlimited self.

I won't claim I'm God, if you won't. But if we don't say it, neither of us is telling the truth. We're taking a crack at expressing our Divinity in the physical—but in unique, totally different ways.

Many energies—including love, growth, healing, intuition— lie beyond the rational mind's ability to understand. The English language has only about eighty-five words for emotions, yet we've all had feelings that we cannot easily define. People in great joy or pain often claim, "I don't have words for this experience."

You are not your thoughts nor your feelings, thank God! You are—thank God again!—a multi-dimensional being, creating your reality at every moment. The discovery of your unique dimensions and their use is the greatest adventure of all!

~ ~ ~

On one level, we're gods. On another level, we're kids. Meanwhile, we're learning the power of our thoughts, on both levels at once! That makes our lives interesting and—all too often— difficult!

The subtle, unseen realms are a natural part of human experience, yet often viewed with skepticism and doubt. To expand your access to energy and increase your power to heal, you must connect with the many dimensions of yourself—and the oneness that pervades all reality. No aspect of reality is outside this Oneness; and every part of it is available to support healing and growth.

~ ~ ~

So powerful are we that we can too easily create the illusion of being separate and lost. The question is not how often you lose contact with your power and divinity, but how can you reconnect with these larger dimensions?

Experiment #47

The "Sweet Influence" of the Pleiades

1. If you're located in the Northern Hemisphere, go outside under a clear autumn/winter sky and find the constellation called the Pleiades, also known as the Seven Sisters.

2. Focus on the pattern of the constellation. Breathe deeply and calm your mind.

    ~ ~ ~

    Then close your eyes.

3. Ask the constellation to send you healing energy.

    Then turn the back of your neck toward the constellation.

4. Imagine the constellation beaming vibrant healing energy—white, or whatever color you prefer—into your seventh cervical vertebra (the bump at the base of your neck). Hold your upper back, neck and medulla oblongata receptive to this energy, visualizing this area being filled with light.

5. Focus in this manner for several minutes, until you feel the flow of energy come to an end. *Give thanks.*

6. Throughout the next several days, whenever you feel any physical or emotional pain, call upon the energy within your seventh cervical vertebra. Direct it to the area of your body requesting healing.

    Again, give thanks.

Welcome to the Discovery Zone!

Anyone who's stopped exploring the unknown in life is heading for the exit.

How many times have you approached a new challenge with a map in your hands, imagining just what you fully expected to encounter? How many times has the unknown failed to match the map, spoiling the whole adventure? Too often we fear the unknown, afraid to explore because "you never know what might go wrong." We often fear the next lesson, because we can imagine the one after that being really ugly.

But healing limitations always involves discovery—the process of stepping into the unknown. *Real* exploration and discovery require that you give up the need to understand. All too many of us use the excuse, "But I don't understand" to avoid facing our fears of the unknown. Understanding will come—in hindsight. It's a gift that you and I can pick up as we exit the Discovery Zone, not one we're handed upon entry.

~ ~ ~

Meanwhile, any journey into the unknown affords a greater experience of your own identity. Consider, for purposes of this exploration, that the only thing you'll even encounter in the unknown is a greater dimension of YOURSELF!

~ ~ ~

Angie, an East Coast client I work with by telephone, was struggling with the unknown of starting a business that followed her passion for teaching art to children. She had spent six years in marketing, and had become very attached to her income and its resultant lifestyle.

"What's in the unknown that you don't want to face," I asked her. "When did the unknown betray you?" In that context, Angie had to concede that she was in the middle of exploring an opportunity to expand her creative expressions, despite her fear of failure and loss of certain comforts.

"I can see how I've always grown in my life," Angie responded, "even when I thought it wasn't possible. Whenever I've stepped into the unknown, all I ever had to do was convince myself that my limitations weren't real."

Angie and I have had several ongoing discussions about what it takes to trust the unknown. Like most of us, Angie won't let herself trust the unknown at those times when she doubts that she's an eternal being—with resources beyond these realms of time and space. As Angie learned to heal her fears, she found a greater ability to trust not only the unknown, but also her passion for teaching children.

Perhaps we've all called the unknown into our lives so that we can better learn trust. Perhaps the discovery of the unknown self is the only path there is—what we've always wanted to do!

~ ~ ~

Could it be, the unknown self is always growing faster than our ability to discover it? Maybe that's the true definition of being eternal.

~ ~ ~

In many Near-Death Experiences, subjects feel that they are in touch with all knowledge. Upon returning to life, these souls report great sadness at having to leave this access to omniscience. Could be we were meant to access this state while alive, and not have to wait until after death. Could the unknown portions of yourself be waiting to support you with access to greater knowledge and intuition, and more effective healing and manifestations?

You may not believe in multiple lifetimes, but most of the world does consider the possibility that we inhabit our physical bodies the way seedlings do pots—whenever we wish to grow, we "transplant" into a new body, with a new set of lessons. To any past lives, add future lives, and lives in alternate universes within the same time continuum, and the possibilities *really* start to open up. It can be fun (or threatening) to wonder if some other dimension of yourself was born as the opposite sex. How would your life be different?

Okay, breathe like a man.

~ ~ ~

Breathe like a woman.

~ ~ ~

Notice how your beliefs produce different experiences by merely changing gender perspectives.

One easy way to explore your unknown dimensions is through the dream state, where most of us have experienced the ability to fly, or enjoy any number of talents and abilities. While performing these wondrous feats, did you have an identity crisis? Of course not! In the dimensions of self we access in dreams, we have no doubts about ourselves being there— it's only to this reality's outer mind that our dreams seem irrelevant. And our dreams often give us notable insight into the challenges we face in this waking dimension.

We've all had moments of intuition and certainty. You and I have both received information and energy without being able to rationally account for the experience. Most likely, these higher dimensions are sending us resources to facilitate the goals we want to live out. And you're meant to consciously use your talents and abilities of self to facilitate growth and healing in these other dimensions, as well.

~ ~ ~

After many years of seeking to nurture my own intuitive skills, I realized that I'd automatically discounted many inner messages, simply because they didn't make sense to my outer mind. As I strove to become more conscious of this automatic mental behavior, I found that hearing these inner, intuitional messages made me want to make different choices.

Early one morning, as I was packing for a 200-mile bike ride, I heard that inner voice say, "Take the black electrical tape." My rational mind immediately countered with, "Why in the world would I need electrical tape on a bike ride?"

I didn't bother trying to answer that question; I simply threw the tape into my pack and forgot about the incident. Nine hours and ninety miles later, as I was parking my bike in a downpour, a complete stranger pedaled up to me and asked, "You wouldn't happen to have any electrical tape, would you?"

I of course remembered that morning's incident, and handed him the tape. He explained that his bicycle seat was coming apart, and he thought that in the rain, electrical tape was the only thing that would effect an emergency repair. That tape was worth its weight in gold, for all the times I've reminded myself that my intuitions don't need to make sense to me right now.

~ ~ ~

While exploring the unknown, it helps to drop your need to understand. Ask questions, yes, but without demanding answers. Keep opening doors to as many options as possible. Don't worry about making major decisions—it's not decision-making time, it's discovery time. Pay attention to your urgings, desires and intuitions. And have fun on the journey!

By identifying with your multi-dimensional self, you no longer need to protect yourself from pain—you're far bigger than it is, and you can claim your birthright of healing. Why bother to build forts against an enemy, when the enemy truly wants to deliver a useful message? And by accepting the possibility of your many dimensions, you can more easily access the present moment, the only place where "superhuman" abilities like telepathy, clairvoyance, and prescience are available.

~ ~ ~

To access your unlimited self, choose healing over protection, acceptance over resistance, and expression over hiding. Again, accept the sacredness of this present moment. Being multidimensional, you have power to free yourself from limitations in any dimension, and can bring to the present any ability you want to express. Why else would Christ and other masters say, "All this that I do, you can do, and more"? Once you accept that the self is vaster than any single dimension, any challenges you face become easier. Remember, problems are simply tools we've constructed to discover ever more of our unknown, multidimensional selves.

~ ~ ~

Whenever I'm facing a challenge, I stop for a moment and imagine a future dimension of myself who's already mastered this particular lesson. Then I ask that facet of myself to help me master this lesson now, giving thanks as I do so.

This works amazingly well. When I'm riding my bicycle up a particularly steep hill, I call on the dimension of myself that's physically very strong, and every time, I experience a noticeable ease in pedaling. I don't think either you or I have much choice about facing challenges. After all, we're creating them! But I know we can discover what it takes for our lessons to be fun. So, experiment!

~ ~ ~

There's no need to manage your growth and evolution. That's being taken care of by a portion of you that's far greater than your conscious, rational mind. This higher dimension speaks to us in our daydreams, as we sleep, in our meditations, and directly through the subconscious.

Your Higher Self is in touch with the full measure of your limitless power. It communicates with all your aspects, all your dimensions. It has a vested interest in expressing its unlimited self through a finite, physical form (you!). Connecting with the Higher Self frees you from any past event where energy stagnates, and where unhealed trauma, limiting beliefs, loss, and pain lead to unwanted behaviors.

Where can you best access your unlimited, Higher Self? Only in the present, our only point of power. You and I cannot communicate with the Higher Self if we're resisting or trying to control our present experience. (Many of us carry the notion that this Higher Self isn't available whenever we're in pain. What silliness!) Acceptance automatically promotes growth, and the Higher Self directs that growth infallibly. Learning to trust this link with the Higher Self brings enormous freedom.

Experiment #49

Connecting with Your Higher Self

1. Sit quietly. Close your eyes. Breathe.

   Simply imagine a connection with an eternal, all-knowing Self.

   ~ ~ ~

2. Once you connect, ask this dimension of yourself to focus its energy at your root chakra—that energy center/vortex between your genitals and anus. Focus on this spot for several minutes, and notice the feelings that you experience.

3. Continue this exercise at the other main energy centers—the sacral chakra (two inches below the navel); the solar plexus; the heart; the throat (at your voice box or Adam's apple); the third eye (center of your brow); and finally at the crown chakra (at the crown—some say slightly *above* the crown—of your head).

4. Spend several minutes experiencing each chakra. Note the sensations of energy in each.

5. Give thanks.

Consciously communicating with the Higher Self is one of the greatest joys of life. Not only can I listen and receive valuable information about current challenges and lessons of my life, but I can ask for specific insights as well. I find it very useful to ask my Higher Self for insights into detoxifying my limiting thoughts, painful emotions and physical limitations. Gandhi once said, "I don't internally cleanse for cleansing's sake, I cleanse so that I may better hear the still, quiet, voice of God Within."

Experiment #51

Getting Advice from Your Higher Self

1. Sit quietly, close your eyes, breathe deeply.

~ ~ ~

Accept your present feelings.

2. Identify a point of clarity you seek in your life.

3. Imagine connecting with your Higher Self or God Within.

4. Ask this spiritual Essence to create a solid communication with your consciousness. (Just seek this link in the present; no need to maintain a permanent link—it's already there).

5. Ask for clarity about the issue you identified in Step #2.

6. Listen. Give up any attachment to consciously hearing an answer now, but do stay receptive for the remainder of your day. Tomorrow morning, explore your dreams for any hints or hunches you may have received.

7. Give thanks.

Don't expect that this dimension of yourself will always communicate verbally, in English. Once, meditating, I asked my

Higher Self this exact question: *Why don't I always get verbal instructions, but receive sensations and insights instead?*

Immediately, I saw a blueprint-like image of a cutaway view of my brain, showing me the path that any verbal message must travel to reach my consciousness. I saw a dot of bright light, traveling a very circuitous path. Then, for comparison, I watched the path of a sensory message, whose shining dot traveled a very direct route. Many messages from my Higher Self come in the form of feelings, which I can then process in a more leisurely time frame. Remember, the ancient Hawaiian Huna system taught that the subconscious mind was the direct line to the Higher Self. Physical sensation is one of subconscious's basic languages, so it makes no sense to deny pain and then expect to be able to access your unlimited dimensions.

Whenever you or I stubbornly refuse to heal past events (by blaming others or declaring ourselves victims), our present lives will reflect limitation and pain. But with the help of our Higher Self, we can heal the past, freeing ourselves from limitations we created long ago.

Experiment #53

Reprogramming "Past" Dimensions

Return to those days of yesteryear!

1. Recall a limitation you believed in as a child, like "I'll never be able to ride this dumb bicycle."

2. In a moment of stillness, mentally show that child a videotape of yourself riding a bicycle effortlessly, joyfully. As your inner child views the video, direct it to breathe.

~ ~ ~

3. Repeat this exercise over three days. You can, in effect, help reprogram your childhood mind so that from that point on, your bicycle riding becomes more enjoyable than ever.

4. Now, go out and start pedaling. Acknowledge any changes in your experience, and give thanks.

(Extra credit for using this exercise with more than *ten childhood limitations!*)

Connecting with past experience releases a great deal of energy and gives you more freedom to use that power. Specifically, connecting with your childhood self lets you reconsider choices made from that limited perspective. Using a more expanded point of view, you can change your life from that moment on—because your past self is only one slim dimension of who You really are. This notion can stimulate a vast array of healing options.

Bless the past, so you can use all the lessons that you've created there!

~ ~ ~

Experiment #55

Asking Your Higher Self to Heal Fears of the Future

1. Sit calmly. Breathe deeply. Close your eyes.

    ~ ~ ~

2. Imagine a movie screen showing a brief film clip from your probable future— about which you feel fear, anxiety or uncertainty. (This event could depict illness, a bad career move, even your death.)

3. As you view this image, fully experience your emotions. Keep consciously breathing.

    ~ ~ ~

4. Feel the energy held within this scene. Ask it to help your Higher Self express itself more completely in this physical realm. Or ask the energy to speed successful completion/resolution of the future event you've imagined.

5. Stay in touch with any feelings until they fade away or disappear. Remember to breathe. Listen for any additional messages. Give thanks.

PART THREE

Healing Your World

CHAPTER ELEVEN
From Scarcity to Abundance:
Wanting, Asking, Manifesting

One of the most captivating experiences of my childhood was a visit to an aviary in nearby Denver. I was in awe at the cacophony of song, the sight of so many birds soaring through a tropical jungle housed within the immense glass structure. I could think of nothing I wanted more in life than my own aviary. But I quickly decided I'd never have the money to build such an edifice. Even if I did, there would be many more worthy causes to spend it on. So I dissuaded myself from my aviary dream. Although it was a rational decision, still I felt like some core joy in my life was forever lost.

One day, decades later, after I'd moved to my Seattle residence, I was watching literally dozens of birds thronging the two feeders I keep in my courtyard. For two years, I'd been hosting birds galore, sharing the joy of their presence with many of my clients. Suddenly it hit me: Here was the aviary I'd wanted as a boy, only this one was better! I didn't have to build a structure to house the birds: They came by my home freely, every day. I could enjoy watching them soar away into the sky, knowing they would return.

For more than 30 years, I'd lost touch with that deeply held childhood desire. Then I reconnected with a childlike joy of living I wasn't even aware that I'd lost. And my open-air aviary offered lots of enjoyment to my clients, nourishing them as well.

This experience has been one of my most dramatic demonstrations of the power of desire, also showing how our thoughts can *impede* the realization of what we truly want.

Many people use energy to manifest scarcity—of money, time, opportunity, and ultimately, love. Since the universe is designed to bless us with abundance, it must take considerable energy to block that flow!

When I tell clients that they're responsible for their own scarcity, they're often amazed: "Who wouldn't love themselves enough to experience abundance?" Yet we often create lack, rather than glimpse our unlimited selves. Ever wonder why so many of us seem to be hiding out behind the excuse, "But I don't know what I want!" Often we don't realize our subconscious attachment to beliefs that manifest as scarcity. For example, we believe that the deep pain of disappointment means that we've failed somehow, or that God is punishing us. Early in life, we decide to avoid this invalidation and the risk of such pain, by simply giving up wanting anything.

The energy contained within such thinking very readily manifests as scarcity.

~ ~ ~

Useful exercise: Identify your top ten disappointments in life. What was the want that was thwarted in each disappointment?

~ ~ ~

For many of us, scarcity can be the best teacher there is, because it reflects some area where our integrity has slipped out of balance, where we've focused on some misconception. Sometimes we believe that we don't deserve what we want. Usually we'll begin examining our self-imposed limitations when scarcity has become a big enough monster that we hear ourselves squeak.

Journal Exploration #57

Healing Scarcity

1. Identify those areas of life where you experience any sort of lack (love, talent, capability, health, money, time, opportunity).

2. In each area, identify past experiences or present beliefs that limit how much you are loved and accepted. Focus on any ideas that tend to diminish your validity in any way.

3. Forgive yourself. Ask your Higher Self to help you love and validate yourself in those areas of your life. Accept all manifestations of scarcity as valid lessons to be learned, on the road to accepting your birthright of abundance.

4. Give thanks.

5. Identify areas of abundance. Again, give thanks. In fact, create a celebration, offering gratitude for abundance in your life.

~ ~ ~

Most of us don't acknowledge our incredible abundance—the abundance of time in our lives, for example. We burn out instead, and then attempt to manage our scarcity of time. We time manage, cut projects short, and shortchange our relationships. Yet, managing scarcity always produces more scarcity (resistance produces persistence). No wonder insurance companies bet that we'll die only two years after we retire!

Are Desires Really Desirable?

Paradoxically, Western culture's emphasis on materialism actually reflects our *resistance* to wants and desires. We view desires as suspect, worrying that unbridled wants will lead us downward into the gutter. (Ever seen that W.C. Fields short, *The Fatal Glass of Beer?*) We fear that passions will rule our lives, replacing our highest potentials with compulsions and addictions. But as I explained to Anne, addictions are just diversions of the energy that is designed to manifest through our unique talents, gifts and potentials. Addictions and dependencies tell us, You're not using enough of yourself.

For years I struggled to quit smoking, convinced I was weak. I told people, "Up in heaven, when they line up the smokers who tried to quit, I'll be at the head of the line of those who failed the most."

In exploring my cravings, I found that underneath them were— surprise! —feelings of loneliness. And from my great teacher, Loneliness, I discovered that I wasn't given the gift of life so that I could waste it waiting for someone else to make me happy. If I can't be happy in this moment now, in these exact circumstances, then I'm focused on a distortion. (Buddha said, "It's no great gift to give a person happiness. The great gift is to help a person learn to heal unhappiness.") The universe is unfolding as it should! My loneliness had been guiding me to recognize and accept the sacredness of this moment, now.

Boy, did my ego need an attitude adjustment when I got that message! But guess what? No more desire for cigarettes. Hmmm!

My cravings also revealed my dependence on excuses. For most of my life, I told myself that healing my tobacco addiction was too great a struggle. One day, I went into my feelings and discovered that underneath all those justifications was simply a desire to love myself more completely—and a fear of failing that!

~ ~ ~

Experiment #59

Accessing Your Addictions' Hidden Message

1. For a three-week period, commit to suspending any judgments about your addiction. During this time, whenever you think about your habit, repeat to yourself, "I am a Divine child of God, with a right to be learning this lesson, in exactly the way I'm learning it." (Remember, acceptance accesses growth and healing.)

2. During this period, locate all sensations in your body associated with the addiction. Feel them.

    ~ ~ ~

    . . . Do the Heal a Hurt exercise (page 72) and the Getting Advice exercise (page 134).

3. Feel for the energy within these feelings and desires. When you connect with that energy, simply ask it to help you grasp whatever greater expression of yourself this addiction is masking. What talents and expressions don't you allow yourself? What is this costing you?

4. Be especially open to feelings of loss, anger, and powerlessness. In short, be prepared to pass through a process of grieving and mourning, because each addiction represents a greater expression of self that you've been denying.

5. Look for ways to give thanks for this lesson. When you release an addiction, tremendous energy becomes available. If you and I didn't have the power

to move through the addiction lesson, humankind would have gone extinct long before now. You will learn more of your power.

6. Should you want to be free of this addiction, begin the process at the time of the new moon. (*See page 94.*)

Louise was deeply frustrated with her failures to curb her addiction to sugar. As we worked together, she discovered her craving was held together by feelings of unworthiness, separation and a childhood belief that she wasn't smart enough for her father to love her. Her true addiction was to this limiting belief! As Louise used her breathing to direct this addiction's energy to help her accept her own value and oneness in her life, she began to notice her sugar cravings diminishing.

In their grappling with wants and desires, too many of my clients rely on a simplistic, drastic rule: Fulfill 'em or kill 'em. If I'm hankering for chocolate, either I should go straight to the candy store *right now*—or else dismiss and reject this desire, possibly forever! Or I can disable my craving by falling asleep and, upon awakening choosing a trendy substitute for chocolate. (Distraction *á la* sex? Shopping? Software?) Or I can self-righteously punish myself for wanting chocolate in the first place. (After all, how can I be so weak, after all these years?)

I can keep denying my desire till I pass a storefront display. Then, I'm a pawn to this monster desire seeking to enslave my salivary glands. Or I can fantasize about my next chocolate experience, asking this hopeful daydream to sustain me through the next few weeks of struggle. (There's something wrong with this picture, and God isn't giggling.)

Often I reject a desire because I can't predict how it will manifest—but this only drains power from my ability to create. Or I kill a desire because I fear it won't be fulfilled, and want to escape disappointment. Ultimately, denying desire leads to the pursuit of empty goals. Killing our desires leads to deep feelings of isolation and confusion: not knowing—or even better, discovering! —what you really DO want.

Lewis Carroll said it best: "Always jam tomorrow, never jam today." Yet I've seen grown men and women build altars to their anticipations, devoting their lives to that sorry worship. If you want to breathe, please do, or you'll suffocate!

~ ~ ~

Self-denial (by which people usually mean denial of temptation) is often considered a noble thing. But I suggest that we're better off accepting our desires, the same as our pains: They're messengers! They contain abundant energy. Without them, how can we access our innate power to manifest what we desire most? The power of desire, I suspect, helps us discover more of our unlimited selves! And whenever we suppress wanting, we block access to our unique potential, and our life's true purpose.

Frank, a client of mine, told me that his business was failing. His receivables weren't being paid, and his front office traffic was down. He was behind on his payroll taxes and planning a second mortgage, juggling creditors and hiding from the taxmen.

"How do you want this situation to resolve?" I asked him.

"I want my business to succeed, of course!" he responded.

"What do you need to do to accomplish that?"

Frank realized that he'd avoided making changes to his staff. He'd been procrastinating about implementing some marketing ideas, had been judging himself a failure and not forgiving himself. I suggested that he start focusing on what he *did* want—and act consistently with that point of view.

In one month's time, Frank's business had turned around!

"Not my Will, but Thine be done?"

Some religions teach us to abandon our individual desires and seek only God's will. But are our wills really separate from God's? If each of us is a unique expression of God, then it follows that our wants and desires must be sacred too! Even when we use our wills in a way that produces pain, we create lessons with the potential to lead us home to our divinity. I've found that many of the people I counsel can go back to the time when they first stopped trusting themselves and the fact that their unique will is a reflection of God's will. They then started shaping wants and desires consistent with comfort and protection from pain. This only led to futile attempts to control their lives, further distancing themselves from the power of their divinity and their birthright of healing.

I'd like to suggest a new way to handle wants and desires. Simply feel them! Accept them as valid sensations, not as decisions.

Experiment #61

Releasing Suppressed Passions and Desires

This is an adaptation of a powerful exercise taught to me by a wonderful healer named Hanna Kroeger.

1. In the course of a quiet evening, write a letter to yourself. Express *ALL* your feelings about the wants, desires, and passions you've been denied (or believe were denied you) in life. Write about the anger, the blame and judgments, disappointments, shame and frustration. Expound on feeling helpless, hopeless and powerless to fulfill your passions. Write about relationships you wanted that others wouldn't join in, toys you couldn't have, contributions you thought you couldn't deliver.

2. Spend no more than one evening on this letter. After you finish it, go to bed and fall asleep.

3. When you wake up, don't read the letter again. Simply burn it.

4. Over the next several days, as memories of this letter return to your consciousness, give thanks for your healing. Dedicate any residual energy to experiencing a wider range of wants and desires, to support your greatest growth and fullest contributions.

~ ~ ~

When someone asks me to justify my desires, I reply, "Isn't my wanting it enough?" Conversely, I believe that my *not* wanting is reason enough for me to forego anything that others want me to do.

Whenever you find yourself becoming critical and complaining, that's a sure indicator that you're not communicating—to yourself and to others—what you truly want. Not only are you in pain, but you're not letting yourself be honest about your own desires. (This insight is very useful when you're facing people who want to attack you!). Discover your true desires, and watch your critical feelings dissipate!

Tiffany came to me, complaining about Pat, her mother-in-law from hell. During one visit, Pat had asked Tiffany and her husband if they would prefer a ham sandwich or chicken salad for lunch. They both said, "chicken salad," at which point Pat erupted, throwing their sandwiches across the kitchen. "You never want to eat my ham sandwiches," she raged.

Tiffany immediately decided never to tell Pat what she really wanted, but instead find out what Pat wanted for her. For years, Tiffany walked on eggshells around Pat, accommodating her every desire. Feeling victimized, she kept trying to fit Pat's expectations, and had deep conflict over their emotional distance. As we worked on her pain, Tiffany discovered that denying the truth of her own wants was producing pain, causing her to withhold love from herself. Through this lesson, Tiffany learned not only that she's the ultimate authority for her own validity, but that she cannot claim her worth without honestly expressing her own wants and desires.

Once she stopped "giving away" her power to Pat, Tiffany's relationship with her mother- in-law became based on honesty, rather than control and domination.

Lots of us no longer experience desires in their true form, because we've devoted too much energy to suppressing them. Identifying them is a highly useful skill.

Experiment #63

Identifying Desires

1. Fast for one day. Drink plenty of non-caffeinated, non-alcoholic drinks, but refrain from eating food.

2. Late in the day, visit a bakery. Inhale the smell of freshly-baked bread and pastries.

3. Notice where the sensations are occurring in your body.

4. Breathe.

~ ~ ~

5. Over the next several days, notice any sensations in the same locations of desire identified during your bakery visit.

6. Once you've identified a similar sensation, ask your body, "What's the want or desire associated with this feeling?" Listen. Watch for symbols of hidden desires in your dreams.

7. Give thanks.

Every desire is a messenger! As you locate its sensation in your body and ask it to deliver its message, suspend the need to make any decisions. Decision-making time will come—later—and will be much easier after you've received the message.

That message may be an idea, a memory, another sensation, or nothing at all. The questions to ask: *Did the messenger go away? Did the desire disappear?* That's how to tell if you've gotten the message. When I go into my sensations about craving chocolate, I discover a great yearning in my mouth and jaws which—when I feel them and ask about their message—reveal that I'm denying feelings of loneliness. Once I let myself feel the loneliness, I discover a still deeper message: that of feeling unfulfilled because I want others to validate me, rather that accepting that job myself.

At this point, I understand that chocolate completely misses what I'm truly wanting.

Experiment #65

Further Exploration of Addiction

1. One day a week, for three weeks, fast from sugar, sweeteners, honey, any refined or natural sugars.

2. Journal the feelings you're aware of during this day. Remember, lots of deep, connected breaths.

    ~ ~ ~

3. Work through any pain using the Heal-a-Hurt exercise, page 72.

4. Ask the energy with any cravings or desires to support you in hearing the messages within all the feelings associated with sugar.

5. Give thanks.

    ~ ~ ~

Our desires indicate how we want to expand our self-expression of ourselves, and our wants point to greater contributions we're eager to make. But what about conflicting desires? Why do attempts to resolve them so often prove disastrous?

Jack, one of my associates, wanted to be in Seattle with his mother and siblings, but also longed to pursue his career in San Diego. He could have used love of family to justify leaving his business—or staying with the business, arguing that his family didn't really care about him all that much. Either decision would have created greater dependency on Jack's being "correct." Thus, he would be in San Diego, justifying his career and feeling guilty about his family. He could have returned to Seattle, and been plagued with doubt about lost business opportunities.

Trying to resolve conflicting desires nurtures dependence on control, not freedom. Result: loss of power and even greater unhappiness. Instead, Jack nurtured both desires. He let himself feel both desires, listening for their mesages. In doing so, he realized ways he'd been withholding himself from both his family and his career.

"In the face of conflicting desires," I suggested, "no decisions need to be made." Jack let himself expand his expressions of caring in both areas, and discovered his family truly supported him in pursing his professional life to the fullest!

To achieve peace in the midst of conflicting desires, I recommend exploring the feelings in your body that you've resisted. Once again, just feel, breathe, and listen for the messages. Do they support a process of germination and growth (as in Jack's case)? Or are you trying to manage those desires through a decision-making process?

Perhaps we're not meant to try to decide between desires, but simply trust the conflict's contributing to a greater awareness, one that may simply be beyond our vision at the moment. Allowing conflicting desires to deliver their messages nurtures freedom, not limitation.

Could it be, your true wants lie beneath the desires you experience? Let's say I desire abundance. I can ask for money until the Fed privatizes. But is it more money that I want, or being able to trust the universe? Will money lead me to heal whatever's blocking my experience of the universe as a loving ally? Perhaps the scarcity I'm experiencing is a lesson to teach me how I focus my thought on lack, rather than on love.

If I'm not listening, I won't hear my desires' messages. That's why I often receive insights about my desires in the shower or while driving—when my mind's not actively engaged, but placid and peaceful enough to hear the answers to my requests.

A question I asked Tiffany and many of my clients is, "Are you willing to heal the fear of having what it is you truly want?" Tiffany had to face her fear of Pat's rage before she could express her desire to honestly relate.

If this were Heaven on Earth, could you allow yourself what you truly want? Pursue your desires as though your God were holding your hand, assuring you that your divinity was never in question. That way, you can also communicate with the energy locked (and stagnant) within any desire and consciously direct it to manifest.

Pursuing what you truly want is an expression of your wholeness—thus, a worthy end in itself! To experience wholeness, you don't need to achieve your goals, only to pursue them fervently, and with honesty and integrity. That's why Joan of Arc, Thomas á Becket, and Thomas More became saints.

Our passions are the beacons that draw to us our greatest potentials!

A Short Dictionary of Hidden Desires

Remember how my craving for chocolate taught me that desires are messengers too, seeking to reveal more of the unlimited, unknown Self? Could be, our cravings and dependencies speak of suppressed talents and gifts we're withholding from the world. Here are some of the actual drives that may underlie various desires and obsessions:

Addiction: Manifestation of the energy of a suppressed talent or contribution.

Attachment to the past: Desire to claim the power to heal guilt; to forgive; to heal fears that the future won't meet your expectations.

Beating up on yourself: Desire to return to growth; to trust that life's lessons are your allies; to accept the power of your thoughts.

Cravings for food/alcohol: Hidden want to experience your power to heal rejection and loneliness; to discover a greater measure of your talents, abilities and validity.

Criticism of others: Desire to discover the validity of what you value most.

Dependence on others' authority: Desire to heal whatever blocks your freedom.

Desire for . . .

   approval: Desire to accept your own uniqueness; to accept your personal expressions of love, in the face of others' negative opinions.

   conflict/domination: Longing to heal the fear that others have the power to invalidate you; to love yourself unconditionally.

   control: Desire to trust your Higher Self or your power to manifest and heal.

death: A deep desire to discover that life loves you, truly and unconditionally. Desire to heal feelings of being nothing. (Also see *pain,* below.)

isolation/hiding from life/others: Desire to heal what blocks your personal power; to accept the joy of your unique contribution and purpose; to heal your fears of separation from God; to connect with your oneness with the universe.

pain: Desire to claim the power to heal; to be at peace with your body as a sacred temple, through which God can manifest.

proving yourself: Desire to accept your validity, sacredness, and uniqueness.

punishing others: Longing to master forgiveness (including yourself), and to heal guilt.

victimhood: Desire to heal pain and lay claim to your own sanctity.

Fixation on the future: Deep desire to trust the power of acceptance; to heal fear of the present moment; to trust that growth is the universe's direction; to forgive past injuries; to love yourself in the midst of lessons.

Material possessions: Longing to heal the fear that your life will make no difference; to heal guilt and self-rejection.

Obsession with money and security: Desire to heal failure, disappointment, and/or scarcity; to accept your worth; to heal the blocks to trusting this as a loving universe; to love yourself.

Obsession with work: Desire to expand the value of your contributions; to experience yourself as valuable and contributing to humankind.

Protection from pain: Wanting the power to heal pain.

Relationship dependencies: Desire to grow in loving yourself, and to express more of that love in your world; to expand the power to validate yourself.

Sugar cravings: Longing to experience the sweetness of life; to heal the fear of its loss.

Suppressed desires/feelings: Wanting to heal the fear of desire; to heal the shame of losing passion in life.

Thrill seeking: Desire to heal whatever blocks your joy of the present moment.

Feel free to add your own interpretations to this list—this is new territory! _____

_____

_____

_____

Presto! Manifesto!

Certain religious and metaphysical philosophies have a tradition that every word contains all the energy it needs to manifest. My aviary manifested only after my resistant thoughts went dormant long enough. If as a boy, I had told myself, "I honestly want an aviary. Getting it can be a contribution to other people, too!" imagine how much faster I could have brought that desire about!

For manifesting your true wants, your ideals and contributions, the basic requirement is simply the ability to ask.

Asking activates the process of creation. Yet most of us make our requests as though they were demands, and *hear* others' requests as though they were demands—as though we have no choice in the matter. Thus, when we don't want to face disappointment and rejection, we try to manipulate people—often implying a threat of punishment if they don't comply.

~ ~ ~

One of my favorite manipulations is, "If you really love me, you'll do what I want." Hogwash! In the vast majority of our relationships, we don't let ourselves get honest about our wants, and don't want to risk disappointment if our requests aren't fulfilled.

To the extent that we coerce others, we find ourselves unable to freely ask for what we want—a curious condition for unlimited beings occupying a loving, abundant universe!

Many of my clients balk at asking for what they want, simply because they can't understand how their requests will be fulfilled. I ask, "Are you willing to disclose what you're afraid of?" Most people who wonder "How?" are learning to trust that the universe truly loves them. They resist the idea that this earthly domain was designed to manifest their wants—fearing failure, loss, and disappointment instead. Others keep asking "Why?," seeking proper justification for their wants. Often these people believe that they simply don't deserve unlimited love. Therefore, the manifestation of their desires comes to a standstill. But they've got good reasons for not having what they want!

We're *always* manifesting, but most of us do it unconsciously, manifesting the programs stored within our subconscious minds. To access our power to create, we must be willing to consciously ask for what we truly want. We've forgotten that the subconscious is designed to be accessible. The subconscious wants to reveal hidden information, and by the simple act of asking, you are focusing energy on a particular inner location, which will ultimately reveal what you seek. With these requests, remember to ask three times, give up expectations about the result, and express gratitude as you await the response.

~ ~ ~

Experiment #67

The Power of Asking

1. Sit quietly. Close your eyes. Relax and begin breathing in a conscious, connected manner.

2. As you breathe, visualize air molecules moving into your lungs. Imagine them very eager to hear—and comply with—your requests.

3. Ask these molecules to help manifest a specific intention (such as completion of a project, your life's purpose, or improvement in a relationship).

4. Visualize your intention coming into form. Notice your feelings—both emotions and sensations. What are they? Feel and listen.

5. Give thanks!

   Variations on step #2: Visualize a night sky full of stars, all anxious to hear and comply. Or, as you exhale, ask the energy within the sun for radiant energy. As you inhale, listen for any messages. Cycle this through ten connected breaths. Note results. Give thanks.

Repeat steps #3 through #5.

When asking, remember to stop asking *why* and *how*—words that only prompt your rational mind to hand you "believable" justifications and rationalizations *not* to pursue what you want.

Simply ask for what you want!

Experiment #69

Exercising Your Power

1. Sit in a quiet place, free from distractions.

2. Identify an intention or desire you wish to manifest.

3. Close your eyes and breathe ten deep breaths.

4. Mentally speak to your body, letting it know you have a request you want it to hear.

5. Imagine all the cells of your body perking up and listening to you.

6. State the intention you wish to manifest.

7. Imagine your body's cells—like a very large audience—taking in your intention.

8. Ask those cells to fully support the manifestation you desire.

9. Give thanks.

10. Over the next seven days, observe the results and look for indications of growth.

Often I ask for something very simple: to find the joy in the present moment. This immeasurably enhances my experience of life's diverse offerings. Often I ask that the universe remove any blocks to the full expression of my divine Self. I can't imagine a more fulfilling request!

Experiment #71

Wielding the Hidden Power in Desire

1. Identify a craving, desire or repetitive behavior from the Dictionary of Hidden Desires, beginning on page 157. Locate the feeling. Accept the sensation. Breathe.

    ~ ~ ~

2. Think of that particular behavior or desire as a messenger. Drop any need to judge yourself for having this experience.

3. What do you truly want? Explore the *real* desire underneath the surface craving.

4. Close your eyes. Imagine yourself touching the energy held within this behavior or desire.

5. Ask this energy to help manifest what you truly want.

6. Give thanks! (*For why, see Chapter 15*).

7. Let it go. Wait three days. Note results!

I often work with these exercises in client sessions.

Ron had been working for years with other counselors on his obsession with proving his abusive father wrong. We explored asking his Higher Self for support in healing this need, and he discovered a deep fear. As Ron went into that feeling and began listening, he discovered that if he forgave his father, he would have to give up many of his self-images.

"My whole life will be wrong!" he exclaimed.

Whenever we ask for support in healing an imbalance, it's a message to the Higher Self that we're ready to move through the lesson. Be prepared for the insights you receive!

~ ~ ~

CHAPTER TWELVE
Conflict and Control

Recognize the emotional baggage you're carrying in relationships with others, and you'll expand your ability to manifest what you truly want.

Every conflict has an infinite number of solutions. But when we're under siege, embroiled in arguments, it's hard to remember all the choices at our disposal.

After experimenting for many years, I've yet to experience a control game that nurtures communication. I'll never forget the time I was slowing down for a stoplight in an intersection, when a driver, with his wife and child in the car, hit my Volvo from behind.

My car was undamaged. But I grabbed my Tai Chi staff from the back seat and walked over to his car for a confrontation. Absurdly, he claimed that *my* driving had caused *him* to rear-end my Volvo. I opted for battle. Deciding to force him to either fight me or slink away, I loudly berated him in front of his family.

"You loser!" I exclaimed. "If you think my stopping at a red light caused you to hit my car, you haven't got a clue!"

"You stupid S.O.B.," was his rejoinder. "You were supposed to go through the light."

I raised my voice, so that his family could hear me: "Would you like to call the cops to see if you're right, you idiot?"

He offered physical violence, if I would only "put down that stick!"

"Take it from me!" I invited him. I made him listen to my tirade until he caved in. He had no choice but to get back in his car and drive away.

Clearly, I'd won! And as I watched him drive off, I felt sick. This man who wanted to attack me verbally—and physically—obviously had great pain. I'd missed the opportunity to support him in his healing. Worse, I'd contributed to his even greater anguish, given the humiliation I'd dumped on him.

I'd chosen to fight just to prove I could win, and felt great remorse at my choice. I definitely didn't experience feeling great or powerful, but small and separate.

To engage in this game of invalidating others, we must get them to play the silly game that each of us is the authority for each other's validity. This way, of course, we inadvertently give them the power to invalidate us! We act as if we really did have the power to make them wrong; as if closing our hearts really makes them feel rejected and abandoned. Closing our hearts produces great pain for *ourselves*; yet still we argue for battle.

~ ~ ~

For me, anger usually helps me avoid feeling powerless. Rather than feel that deeper pain, I rage, intimidate, and dominate.

I've heard medical doctors claim that suppressed anger is the main cause of illness. Of course, anger is taboo in many circles, because people assume it's "bad," that there's no way to express it except through attacking and belittling. But if accessing our true power means we need to accept whatever's in the present moment, then anger must be validated too. And I've seen many ways of expressing anger respectfully, so that the message is delivered and healing occurs. If you're at a loss about how to express your anger safely, simply rage with a pillow over your face, and see how quickly you discover the distortion that created the anger.

~ ~ ~

To avoid getting stuck in anger, I go to people I've dumped on and apologize. In doing so, I've had to take ownership of the assumptions and expectations I have about others.

Remember the altercation I had with my father over his hunting dog, Freckles? I assumed he thought I was stupid, that he was trying to control me. He thought he was simply informing me about the dog's idiosyncrasies, and that I was being disrespectful. Cleaning up my anger helps me listen more closely to what others are saying, while imposing fewer definitions on them.

"Whenever two or more are gathered together" in human relationships, there's a powerful opportunity for directing energy, aligning intentions, and manifesting common goals. But when people try to control, manipulate and attack each other, relationships can't effectively access that dynamic power to create what's wanted.

~ ~ ~

Clients ask me how they can reclaim their power. They protest loudly when I suggest they give up the right to do battle—including the rights to judge, blame, punish, and condemn—and then focus on seeing their attackers as divine.

"Giving up my right to battle means giving away my power," they tell me. "No," is my response, "all you'll be abandoning is your need to dominate and control. Giving up the need to invalidate those who attack you is a great way to reclaim your personal power and access creative energy for conscious manifestation." To those who still protest giving up the right to battle, I continue: "How did you feel, the last time you attacked someone?"

Their answer is invariably the same: "I was upset, afraid, and in pain."

"And how did you relate to that pain? Did you accept the pain, or resist it?"

Again, invariably, people realize they believed they were unable to heal their pain, and that their attacks were an attempt to blame, or dump, the pain on someone else.

At this point, the light dawns, and my clients can begin to see that all the people who have attacked them were simply souls in pain who didn't know they could heal themselves, and were trying to control that pain by attacking someone else! As we seek to control our own pain, we will seek to control our bodies, our lives and other relationships as well.

I point out that power is not control. Control is the attempt to force an action, without regard for our own or another's freedom to choose. We assume that if we can control the circumstances around us, then life will manifest what we want. This never works! At best, we've simply intimidated our environment to coddle to our wishes and do our will—and then, for only the short term.

A further "fix" is soon needed. So, in trying to control our own pain, we become highly skilled at domination, intimidation, invalidation, criticism, creating dependencies, and playing "poor me." We withdraw, close our hearts, take our marbles and go home. Seeking to force our agendas on others, we mistakenly believe we have the right to punish each other—and whenever we're trying to avoid (read "control, rather than heal") pain, we automatically revert to these controlling behaviors.

If this sounds like a frenetic sporting event rather than a relationship, you're right. And no one is giggling about it. In trying to impose control, we've impeded our own life's expansion—and we're stuck.

True power is the ability to manifest your intentions, which must begin with accepting things just as they are. Control is based in resistance, power in acceptance—so in actuality, the two are diametrically opposed. Control is restrictive, power is creative.

In order to claim power, give up controlling your physical experiences. Then accept the responsibility of choosing your thoughts, and you can take the lead in creating your own life.

~ ~ ~

As a teenager, when I was having an argument, one of my most self-sabotaging behaviors was to put myself down and agree with my attackers. I blamed myself for their upsets, and felt too stunned to speak up for my wants. It seemed easier—wouldn't speaking up for myself only inflame the conflict? Only after recognizing how I treated myself in a conflict, was I able to start making different choices.

I used to believe that in relating to others, I couldn't always be honest about my wants and desires. Simply by not intruding—not expressing what I truly wanted, but instead trying to please others—I thought I'd be accepted and ultimately, happy in life. I hadn't stopped to realize that I couldn't be to blame for their feelings—I wasn't making their choices about their thoughts. So for many years, I structured my wants and desires to fit others' expectations.

One day, looking at a tree outside my window, I realized that tree had never asked for my permission before growing new limbs and leaves in every direction. The tree was intruding joyfully into its surrounding space, as if fully expecting life to appreciate all its expressions, even the intrusive ones. Examining my beliefs about my right to intrude, I realized that they were based on the fundamental notion that the universe did not accept me exactly as I am. Yet the air has always been there when I've wanted to breathe. Never has the earth not risen to meet my step. Like every other unique form of life, I intrude by my very acts of living.

"To thy own self be true," the powerful admonition that Shakespeare put in Polonius's mouth, could be restated as, "Honoring your validity is a requirement for the effective use of energy." If I can't be honest about my wants and desires, I block my ability to grow. I can't integrate my own present experience and thus, divorce myself from my only point of power, blocking the effectiveness of my creative manifestations. So nowadays, I give myself full permission to intrude—with a deep passion that acknowledges the sacredness of all life around me.

~~~

Competition is great on the tennis court and the chessboard, but I think it's a lousy way of resolving conflicts. Win/lose has never nurtured long-term relationships (which, by the way, is what we're constantly striving to establish with life, our environment, and the rest of humankind).

As I said, I've often gone into battle to prove that others can't control me. It took me long years to realize that by resisting control, I was actually giving away my different options. A great illustration of this is a therapeutic exercise played by two people. One commands, "Stand up," or "Sit down." The other person must do the opposite of what the commander says. It's a dramatic way to demonstrate that when people resist being controlled, they're still far from free.

~ ~ ~

Again, battle is based on the falsehood that others can really invalidate or diminish us. Once you've claimed ultimate authority for your own validity (that is, for loving yourself), no one else has any power to take it away. You simply refuse to believe their point of view! At that point, you can see their controlling behavior as attempts to avoid their own pain—a signal that they're resisting their own experience, often ignorant of their power to heal. Whenever we refuse to sell out our validity to another, we are actually empowering them. We are presenting them with the opportunity to look at their pain as their own creation, rather than continuing to blame us!

~ ~ ~

Now, when I'm faced with someone trying to control me, I determine if they want to communicate, or simply battle. I begin by taking deep, connected breaths. If they want to fight, walking away—withdrawing—has served me best. I let my adversarial wannabes know that I'll be back when they want to talk. When their only goal is Invalidate Ned, I clearly let them know there are other games I'd rather be playing.

Should they *demand* that I stay and fight, I remind them that I'm still the one making choices in my life. Sometimes controllers justify their desire to argue by claiming they have something important to tell me. Now, I am very willing to hear others' feedback, but not delivered on the head of a cudgel!

To find out if my would-be enemies *really* want to talk (while they're demonstrating their latest fighting techniques), I ask them, "Would you mind telling me what's bothering you? How are you feeling?"

If they give me still more blame and judgment, then I leave the field. However, if they look inside, seeking to explore their pain, I *listen*.

Do I try to solve their problems? No! Make them feel better? No! I just listen, sending a message that I accept them just as they are, with whatever experience they're having. I grunt "Un-hunh!"— or perhaps just repeat the emotional content of what they say, without judging it. My intention is that they get the message that by simply accepting their own pain, they'll automatically begin moving through it. At times we men automatically become defensive during conflict, because we believe that doing so validates our manhood. What we're really wanting is to be heard and reminded of the job of validating ourselves.

As we undertake this process of communication during pain, our conflict reveals to me a greater awareness of how my adversary and I reflect each other, what we mean to each other. Conflict is just another messenger, warning that we've resisted growing in a relationship—no matter how brief that interchange may be!

If we employed the same discipline in communicating that we use in fighting, we'd experience Heaven on Earth.

~ ~ ~

Whenever you opt for control, you get stuck.
Accept the conflict, you heal the pain and grow.

Hidden Energies in Honest Expression

In a world that looks to others for validation, warfare is believed to be the final solution to conflict. But those who have been in battle know that no one really wins, because the cost to humanity is too high. Whenever we remember that conflict is truly an opportunity for communication, rather than battle, we again realize that every conflict has an infinite number of solutions—which, as I've said, is hard to remember when we're under siege.

When we fall into conflict, our society trains us to seek control—the implicit promise being that successful control will assure victory.

Clearly, we'll never control ourselves out of being controllers. But in accepting and loving yourself as you learn, you'll automatically grow through the need to control. Choosing to accept yourself in the present accesses greater creative energy, dynamically restoring your relationships. (Imagine what an attitude of self-invalidation does to the quality of our communications!)

Permission to intrude? Granted! Identify your wants and desires. Make mistakes doing so, and clean up any messes you create, in a way that expands love on this planet.

Permission to desire? Granted! Permission to dream? Granted! Permission to freely express your unique blend of talents, abilities and potentials? Granted!

~ ~ ~

Experiment #73

Revealing Your Personal Control Headlines

1. When you seek to dominate your own pain, what do you say to your body? (For example, "I won't feel this," or "This pain isn't so bad.")

    1A. When you seek to dominate other people, what do you say to them?

2. When you seek to invalidate your own feelings, what do you say to your body? (For example, "You're weak, wrong, flawed.")

    2A. When you seek to invalidate others, what do you say to them?

3. When you hold yourself as a victim to your body, and/or your pain, what do you say to your body? (For example, "You are non-responsive, hostile, uncaring and capricious.")

    3A. When you hold yourself as a victim to another, what do you say to them?

4. Share these headlines with those people you've sought to control.

    4A. Notice how readily you become aware of the pain you've sought to hide through your controlling behaviors.

    4B. Is there a subconscious want or desire hidden within the control game?

5. Use any of the healing exercises in this book to help you in getting the messages your pain or hidden desire seeks to deliver.

6. Give thanks.

CHAPTER THIRTEEN
Your Ideal for Humankind and Unique Contribution

Publications like *Forbes*, *Money*, and *The Wall Street Journal* would have you believe that the goal of life is wealth and financial abundance. As an unfortunate result, people pursue money with the assumption that it'll fill all the potholes and sinkholes in their lives.

Many people are pursuing their careers with passion, but don't seem to be having much fun doing it. Successful people often seem to sell out their joy of living in return for their thirty pieces of silver. Successful clients are forever telling me that they can't have what they want because their jobs don't give them time to pursue it. This may be heresy, but I don't think success was to be at the sacrifice of our well-being. Perhaps the true meaning of "work" is really "love in action."

Journal Exploration #75

The Hidden Energy in Time

1. Reduce your working hours one to two hours per day, for three weeks. During this period, you'll be working from five to ten fewer hours per week. List what you would love to do with this extra time.

2. At the end of each week, record three ways your life has changed as a result.

3. At the end of three weeks, ask yourself: Would you like to return to your previous schedule?

~ ~ ~

When used to express love, sacrifice can accomplish a great deal. When used to justify limitation or prove validity, sacrifice only establishes a pattern of growing pain. Think of a single dad who gives up time every night to read stories to his 5-year-old daughter. The time he sacrifices now will propel her into reading on her own, later on.

Caution: Will your sacrifice nurture growth and a greater expression of love? If you aren't loving yourself, but rather just proving that you're a good martyr, it won't be. (*Eager to sacrifice something? See box for suggestions.*)

Thoughts Worth Sacrificing
1. Limitation, judgment, and punishment.
2. Invalidation of your wants, desires and/or lessons.
3. Doubts about your gifts, your talents, and your abilities.
4. Beliefs that you are in any way separate from the incredible lovingness pervading the universe.

Still feel an inclination to renounce something? Ask that impulse's energy to boost your ability to love yourself.

And others! Watch how what you seek to remove from your life *gently withdraws and disappears.*

Most children are in touch with their own unique vision for humankind. They know what they want to be when they grow up, and what they want to do. More often than not, their chosen roles emphasize service to others. Little boys want to be Superman or Batman, a fireman or a Texas Ranger. Little girls want to nurture in their own way . . . as doctors, nurses, teachers and mommies.

You and I arrived on this planet with an ideal for humankind. Some would call this "our purpose," others might term it "a passion to contribute." But in any case, each of us holds, deep in our hearts, a vision of the unique gift we can make to human evolution. I suggest that the whole purpose of freedom and free will is to pursue this ideal, which each of us holds for humankind. Given your unique gifts and talents, no other being on the planet can accomplish that the way you can.

My advice?

Pursue relentlessly whatever ideal you hold for humanity!

Karl, a client, told me that starting when he was seven years old, he'd wanted everyone on earth to know there is a Santa Claus. As he grew up, Karl was distracted by marriages and his pursuit of new careers. By the time he walked into my office, Karl was middle-aged, successful and a survivor of open-heart surgery. He still believed—passionately! —that people deserve to be treated with greater compassion, as though each day were Christmas. But Karl's professional stature prevented his expressing that. He felt lost. And his frustration was costing him his happiness and his health.

Here's the paradox:

While you hesitate to pursue your unique ideal, the world hungers for it.

And you are not required to complete your lessons before you begin pursuing this ideal!

Journal Exploration #77

1. What expressions and desires to give are you
denying yourself?

2. If this were the day of your death, how would you
have wanted to have lived your life?

~ ~ ~

To pursue your ideals freely, you must be honest, emotionally
and intellectually—realizing that your pains, your wants, and your
desires are all valid.

Your loves and joys, your pains and sorrows all point in the
direction of your unique purpose—the great contribution each of
us seeks to make, throughout our lives. To clients who protest, "I
don't know what my purpose is," I reply, "Make your purpose be to
discover your purpose, and don't give up. Listen to your wants and
desires, listen to what's happening in your body. Take on the job of
healing any fear of your purpose."

~ ~ ~

Your purpose is pursuing *you* just as avidly as you are pursuing
it. Silkworms don't know they are weaving the fiber of your clothes,
yet they weave their cocoons with great joy and abandon. When
you've discovered your purpose, you'll know it. Every cell in your
body will know it. All the events of your life will suddenly make
sense, and you'll see how every choice you've made has been leading
you toward the expression of this purpose.

Everything you've done in life has been toward the pursuit of this ideal. Either you're in joy because you're contributing to it, or in pain because you're not.

(*Reread this paragraph!*)

~~~

It took me many years to realize that my life is about helping others know their own divine selves more fully. Looking back, it should have been obvious: My early religious life thrilled me with the promise of a relationship with the Eternal. Later, I was nurtured by the idea that each of us creates our own religion, and the earliest trauma I can remember was having to stay at home one Sunday with my mother, while my father and older sister went to church.

My greatest passion, I discovered, was also my ideal: To rekindle my relationship with the Unlimited Self within, and to support others in that same discovery; to give love, especially where it seems to be lacking. I can't control my ideal; I can only allow it to lead me. I can control my thoughts and accept my experiences, but must bow to my own desire to contribute. In discovering an ideal bigger than my life, I trust that it will guide me without fail. Then I can use the abundant energy surrounding me to support the greater expression of my ideal.

Journal Exploration #79

Discovering Your Purpose

Imagine you win a $125 million lottery! Then you spend ten years traveling, buying resort homes, and spending; and devote the next ten years giving to philanthropic causes. You've rested and retailed yourself into boredom. You're 57 years old. You're healthy. You have $99,000,000 left.

~ ~ ~

Ask yourself . . .

1.   How would you love to see humanity grow? What would you do with your abundance?

2.   List ten things you could do to further human evolution.

3.   If you could manifest anything in support of humankind, what would it be?

Over three consecutive days, spend some time writing down whatever whimsical, serious, outrageous, unthinkable responses you come up with to this question.

A further exercise that supports the exploration of purpose is to write a letter to humankind, acknowledging yourself as unique and expressing what you want to contribute and create.

What do you want to give to us all?

Experiment #81

Using Energy to Support Your Ideal

1. Repeat Experiment #7, pg. 43, substituting the unique ideal you've identified from Journal Exploration #79, pg. 182. Focus on your ideal for humankind. If you don't yet know it, focus on your desire to discover this ideal.

2. Connect with a time you felt passionate in life— perhaps a time of deep inspiration, or even a time of passionate anger.

3. Locate that feeling of passion in your body. Breathe. Ask the energy within that passion to dedicate itself to fully manifesting your ideal.

4. Give thanks. Over the next seven days, observe the results.

Your purpose must be something grand, bigger than life, which your rational mind tells you is impossible. Your ideal *should* look impossible! It should take 30 lifetimes to complete! Rationally, you'll expect the world to castigate you for entertaining such a hope. But pursuing your purpose, you're in touch with the happiness of being on your journey, with little care for the outcome. This pursuit holds within it the greatest amount of energy, for it always evolves the fullest expression of your unique, unlimited self. *This* is happiness.

~ ~ ~

Discovering your true purpose shouldn't be a struggle. Yes, we need to meet the challenges that help us discover our power and strength. But can you meet challenges, and still dedicate your thoughts to the greater expression of your purpose? That deep passion may have been with you for lifetimes, thwarted.

~ ~ ~

As you pursue your passion to contribute, count on making mistakes! Expect failures! Be assured, your ideal will train you to use mistakes to support its manifestation. Your ideal will train you to maintain your focus on your own sacredness, as well as on the gifts and contributions you wish to make.

~ ~ ~

Experiment with that idea and note the results!

What if you recklessly pursue your ideal for humankind? Many of us would use this notion to justify abandoning our ideal, fearing that others will abandon us. We're afraid we'll wind up in trouble! History provides many cautionary examples (Joan of Arc, Davy Crockett, Madame Curie, Father Damian—and Jesus, of course!), to reinforce our worries. But Seth, the entity channeled through Jane Roberts, exhorts us to pursue this ideal recklessly, for it will never betray us. If we pursue it tenuously, however, it will always produce pain.

Most of us, I suspect, *would* die for our ideals, if convinced that sacrifice really would advance our best hopes for human evolution. But the greatest challenges (and thus, our deepest fears) come from *claiming authority* for our own unique ideals.

A very capable woman named Maggie came to see me because she wasn't fulfilled in her career as administrator for a high-flying legal firm. She related a belief she had nurtured as a child: Her family was poor and thus, not acceptable.

During her early years in school, Maggie had withheld herself from classmates. Later on, she began isolating herself from society, justifying her seclusion with continued feelings of unworthiness. Maggie even went the next step in denying her pain by believing, that she didn't need people in order to be happy.

As we untangled her pain and limiting beliefs, Maggie hit a great wall of sadness as she realized her childhood decision had kept her from her opportunity to pursue her unique ideal for humankind. She felt she had lost that deep passion to use her heartfelt desires to contribute. As Maggie let herself heal, she began putting offers on retail fashion boutiques, and today takes great joy in simply sharing herself as customers come through her front door.

Our greatest fears are of failing our potentials and losing the opportunity to pursue our unique ideals. We fear failing at what we'd most love to do, and all too often, we don't let ourselves pursue that contribution. We fear being ridiculed, having our contribution rejected by the world.

Two simple exercises to heal these fears: First, connect with the energy within your fear and ask it to support the fullest manifestation of your contribution. Second, ask yourself, "Can I be counted on to love myself, even if I were to fail at what I'd most love to do?" Breathing helps!

~ ~ ~

Is it frightening to be in charge of our ideals for humanity? Sure! Especially when most people around us are denying their own authority, their own leadership.

But pursue an ideal half-heartedly, and you can't pursue it fervently, joyously! In your personal life, you are the ultimate authority. Your relationships with others must reflect your ideal. If they want to assist in your pursuit, fine! Meanwhile, pursue your unique vision for human growth. Even if it means dressing up in a red, furry outfit during the holidays and sitting in the mall with kids on your lap, *DO IT!*

Pursuing your ideal accesses all manner of energy . . . beyond your wildest imaginings!

CHAPTER FOURTEEN
Listening, Loving, and Learning

One day, getting lunch at the counter of a buffet-style restaurant, I heard a child scream.

Across the room, a man and his son were seated at a table, the boy howling as his father was about to take another swing at him with a dog leash.

Everyone else in the restaurant was trying to ignore the incident. I grabbed my tray and hurried for their table—fearful at first, not knowing what to do.

I stood there until the man looked up. "Looks like you're having a rough time," I sympathized. From the tone of my voice, this guy knew I wasn't threatening him.

I'll call him Howie. Inviting me to sit down, he confessed that he'd lost his job. His wife had just driven their broken-down car to a garage, along with the last of their cash. For him, the last straw had been here at the restaurant, when his son didn't want to eat his food—the last meal that they could afford, till God only knew when.

Listening, I realized that Howie just needed to be heard, not judged or convicted. As he told me his story, I said very little, simply offering a message of acceptance and validation. By that time, he'd released a good deal of his stress and terror. Our short time together left Howie apologetic toward his son—and much more optimistic about his future (with very little prompting from me).

Listening means hearing another's point of view, without fearing that it will undermine your own position. It's not about agreeing or disagreeing. Listening is about accepting their point of view as valid *for them*—right where they are, in the midst of their lessons.

There's tremendous power in listening, without letting your outer, rational mind judge—in part because you'll automatically attract people who can best teach you about yourself. Evaluate your reactions as you listen to others, and you'll gain a wealth of insight into your hidden needs and personal growth.

Choosing to Listen Releases Energy

In my first few years as a therapist, I arrogantly expected clients to listen to *me*—without realizing the profound gift I was demanding!   Listening must be voluntary, and freely offered. Whenever I felt *obligated* to listen to their pain, the clients failed to heal and remained stuck, often compounding the problem by seeing me as the bad guy.

Now, working with my clients, I send them messages of acceptance as I listen. When they complain about their unworthiness, I don't try to change that point of view. Instead, I let them know I've heard what they're saying. I emphasize that I not only consider them valid, but also consider valid the lesson they're in the middle of, regardless of their self-judgment or their pain.

This makes their task of moving through pain much easier— remember, acceptance automatically accesses growth and healing. When clients hear that I accept them just as they are, they find the job of accepting themselves much easier. Listening helps them step into a new awareness, opening up to unseen realms. And out of the unknown, they can access abilities to deal with whatever experience they're creating.

~ ~ ~

Another wonderful thing about listening, which my clients have taught me: When people experience being *heard*, they don't need to defend themselves. They're able to direct energy in creative directions, instead of doing battle. As an added bonus, whenever people experience being heard, they automatically open up their ears, hearts, and minds to new information. (It would be useful to tattoo this mantra on your grey cells also!)

~ ~ ~

Listening magnifies—and multiplies—your personal energy, promoting your *own* healing and growth. Yet whenever anyone has required me to listen on demand, I can hear only my own resentment. Whenever you're not open to listening, just let the speakers know you'll get back to them later. You've just stoppered a major cause of your energy being drained! As you grow in trusting your choice to listen to others, you'll begin to "hear" what your own Higher Self wants to express. The outer mind becomes trained to serve your higher dimensions, not merely the time-and-space ones. You develop the mental calm that allows that still, quiet voice to be heard, rather than having to rely on the Mack-Truck messages that inundate us and threaten to drive us into the ditch!

~ ~ ~

The subtle realms are called that for a reason! And without access to those realms, without listening to yourself, how can you determine if energy is flowing or stagnant?

Listening is intimately linked to asking, which activates both the subconscious and the Higher Self to select information and deliver it to consciousness. In this way, each of us can expand our own gifts of intuition, insight and vision.

Whenever you ask someone to listen to you, greater intimacy develops, even when your listener disagrees. Sharing information lets us manifest things synergistically, in concert with one another, taking advantage of the energy to create that's inherent in relationships. Listening lets us point our mutual goals in the same direction—so we can fit them through the door at the same time. (Again, this requires the risky willingness to honor your own and others' uniqueness, no matter what.) Our wants and desires don't have to agree for creation to occur!

Helpful hint: Whenever you begin to listen, also begin deep, connected breathing at the same time. Whenever you find yourself becoming defensive or getting sucked into someone else's point of view, begin connected breathing to remind you that your listening is a choice. Listen especially to your feelings that are being triggered. Let your Unlimited Self breathe! Notice how that feels!!

~ ~ ~

While We're At It—A Few Notes On Love

We're all here on earth to learn the myriad lessons of love. (Admittedly, terrorists and serial killers might need to learn more than the average person on the street.) Could be, we all secretly love each other, but are overly concerned with embarrassment. Perhaps we're discovering our great passion to love, in part by learning the futility of trying to control love.

I've watched myself get angry at love, believing it's failed me because it hasn't fit my expectations. Then I've closed my heart, rather than learn to let go of my pictures of what love should be. There's great value in learning to serve love as our master and let it guide us to a more powerful expression of our unlimited selves.

~ ~ ~

At every moment, you and I can choose to love ourselves—which is the prerequisite to giving love anywhere else. But that means constantly renewing that choice, even when we're hurting! (Extra credit if you'll allow yourself to do this in front of others!)

~ ~ ~

Loving ourselves is aligned with seeing ourselves as sacred, even while experiencing limitation, pain and conflict. Thus I define *love* as choosing to perceive someone—yourself or another—as unlimited, multidimensional and divine. Yes, this definition is shaky and inadequate, but good enough for this present exploration.

No, loving yourself is not the same as indulging yourself—though this is how most of us think about self-love. Loving ourselves, by the very definition of love, must include those times of failure, pain, and distress. It's no great trick to love the lovely!

Ward, a very successful software programmer, could trace much of his unhappiness to a childhood belief that he was supposed to know how to do things—that being taught somehow proved him stupid. "I want to have a family," Ward explained, "but I don't know how to get into a meaningful relationship."

Early in life, Ward had begun withholding love from himself, not recognizing he was in the middle of learning to love himself. As we worked, he experimented with asking his Higher Self to help him learn to love himself, with fantastic results. Suddenly, friends were introducing him to potential partners.

"Ward," I told him, "You were never meant to learn how to love yourself on your own." All too many of us buy the fallacy that the job should be done all alone. In loving ourselves, we must drop our judgments, accept our feelings as messengers, our experiences as valid, and be willing to discover our unique talents, gifts and potentials—our passion to contribute. It helps to refuse to sell out our oneness with God. The universe is unfolding at every moment to help us learn this lesson!

~ ~ ~

Two-Week Experiment #83

Expanding Your Love for Yourself

1.   For two weeks, increase by a factor of ten the number of times you take a moment during the day to acknowledge your own sacredness.

2.   During this period, notice how the world appreciates you.

3.   Give thanks.

I used to operate on a very nasty falsehood: *I can't love myself unless someone loves me first.* In other words, "I must be loved BEFORE I'm worthy of love."

I'm sure you see the trap! Giving away my authority this way meant creating emotional dependence—an illusion, but one of the worst, as illusions go. I considered others' love for me to be the source of my validity.

Do I need *you* to make *me* feel loved? If so, then whenever I feel "bad," you're not doing your job!

~ ~ ~

This misconception hindered me in any number of ways. Sometimes, I tried to love others while disregarding the job of loving myself—producing pain. One of my greatest fears was that there would be no one with whom I could share my passion to love. Trying to control this fear shaped all my relationships. As you might expect, I chose people who were unavailable—to me, anyway. As I healed this fear and grew in loving myself, it was quite a shock to discover that an abundance of people joyfully welcomed my sharing. As I began more openly expressing love, sometimes in just small, silly ways, a whole new dimension of energy opened up.

Guess what?

Giving love without asking for reciprocation expanded my own willingness to love. I take great comfort in the lesson that, even in those moments of joy when I'm alone, I can ask the energy of that experience to infuse with love the universe around me.

~~~

Never assign the job of loving yourself to others, because it's not a job to be delegated. It's not others' fault when they fail at the job that only you (and God) can perform effectively. This doesn't mean we're not loved, simply that others' love isn't the source of our being loved.

Some of us believe that giving love is the same as receiving it: I love you, thus you must love me. Thus, when others impose love on you, it becomes an obligation, not a freely given expression. Yet, we must be free to do both—give and receive. That means we cannot impose our love on another, or else we've empowered yet another silly control game.

Yes, there's a downside risk. Freeing yourself from emotional dependency is so disruptive that relationships often change—or break up! But again, any resulting pain is meager, compared to the effort of trying to force others' love for the rest of your life. Consider: if we pursue this ideal of loving tentatively, it will always produce pain; but if we pursue it recklessly, it will never betray us!

I've learned something about dependency by watching the birds outside my office window. Adult birds will bring their fledglings to the feeders, where their offspring will perch on a tray full of seeds, screaming to be fed. The parents struggle to feed their young, trying to teach them that's food they're standing on. It's fascinating to witness the moment when the young birds suddenly expand their awareness and give up their dependence on their parents.

One day, I was looking out the window at the feeder, watching a young fledgling sparrow beginning to feed himself, when its mother flew in and interrupted him, trying to force food into its beak. I realized that dependency can run both ways, that in some relationships, both parties need to change their thinking.

Many people seek sympathy, confusing it with compassion—as if the extent of another's sympathy is the measure of their love. But examine the sympathetic response! Does it see others as capable and unlimited, creating the circumstances of their lives as opportunities to discover more greatness? By demanding sympathy, I try to prove to myself that I'm lovable—thus mirroring my belief that I'm not.

The opportunity to love is never denied you, save by your own limiting beliefs. But to discover how to express love right now, you must be willing to accept the present. And too often, the expressions of love aimed your way right now don't match your expectations of how you're supposed to be validated and cherished and gratified. Too often, you and I define how others should love us, believing that our own expressions of love are the standard and the norm.

To prove our validity, we ask others to agree with our self-image. When they don't, we call them wrong and try to control them—

get them back in line. But whenever you depend on others to prove that you're loveable, you're not taking responsibility for your own withheld love—which produces its own punishment. I've seen countless conflicts borne out of the blame we assign each other for the pain of withholding our own love!

~ ~ ~

If this is a lesson you're facing, please refrain from invalidating yourself here. Each one of us has failed in many ways to express love to the full extent we are able. But by learning to love the aspects of yourself that have withheld love, you free yourself from the stagnation of the blame game. You expand your ability to forgive those who withhold love from you. If any choice costs us our freedom to love, that choice will cost us our birthright of abundance, health, and happiness as well.

Journal Exploration #85

1. Identify the areas of life where you withheld love from yourself.

2. Identify the areas of life where you withheld love from others.

3. Identify your pain when you withhold love. Who are you blaming for these feelings?

4. Forgive yourself—and others—for any love withheld.

~ ~ ~

Could be, this universe is teaching us to love.

Could be, the greatest door to energy and healing is through willingness to love—despite the rational mind's judging, disliking, and diminishing.

Could be, the only pain we've ever created for ourselves arose from withholding love's expressions.

Could be, the fundamental truth of every human relationship is that we truly love each other, and are passionately eager to express it.

Lessons and How to Recognize Them

Pretend that you're an Ascended Master, creating each moment of your life. You are a "location" where God manifests, in unique form. You've returned to earth simply to learn some lessons about your Unlimited Self. You are both your own teacher, and your own student.

For you, even painful events are opportunities. You're always drawing just the lesson you need for your next expansion of consciousness. Having mastered many lessons, you have a deep passion to master the ones facing you now.

We often cherish the misperception that our worth is somehow proved or disproved by the lessons we're assigned. Back in high school, no one wanted to be left back and have to repeat a grade— and so, we often believe it's shameful to have to repeat a lesson— especially a "bad" one, like alcoholism or mental illness. But there's really no shame in repeating real-life lessons: that's called practice! We all keep repeating a variety of lessons, until we discover greater measures of ourselves within the lesson.

~ ~ ~

Consider any lessons you've resisted or ignored: Have they really disappeared? If you've spent any time on this planet, you've discovered that resisting lessons only helps them persist—which means you get to repeat them! And because the choice is always yours, you can make your lessons fun, or a struggle.

What if you don't like the current lesson? Arguing that your present moment isn't unfolding as it ought to just creates drama around the lesson. Great entertainment, but no learning takes place.

We've often judged others as wrong because of the lessons they've taken on—not realizing that each of us is working on just the right curriculum. All of us would prefer that our neighbors were learning to walk on water. However, no one ever crosses our path whose particular current lesson doesn't somehow have a gift for us.

~ ~ ~

I find it useful to think that all of my challenges are lessons I've borrowed from the great Lesson Lending Library. None of these lessons is really mine; they're just on loan until I master them. Each and every one of them wants to show me more of myself and help me recover the joy of growing, so that I can expand the expressions of my ideal for humankind.

Probably every lesson from the Library contains another opportunity to further our abilities as powerful, creative beings, tapping into unlimited energy. Not one of them—including our greatest addictions and obsessions—are bigger than our ability to move through them and learn from them. Those who already checked out the same lesson before have made my learning a little bit easier, through their efforts in learning it. If you pick up one of the lessons I've worked on, perhaps you'll find it easier than I did. And may other people be hastened in their growth, simply by hearing about *your* learning.

CHAPTER FIFTEEN
Forgiveness, Trust and Blessing

If you're hurting, blaming, or seeking revenge for *any* painful event, then a portion of your awareness—and the energy that goes with it—is useless, locked away in the past. By forgiving and releasing that past event (that is, accepting its validity), you free yourself to operate in the limitless here and now.

We learn funny misconceptions about forgiving. For example: *If I get punished enough, then I've got permission to forgive myself.* And: *If I punish you enough, then I can forgive you. I might forgive, but I'll never forget.* These notions are intimately linked with the self-contempt that's so endemic in our society.

We build our own self-contempt whenever we invalidate our own experience.

If you operate this way, I bet you'll find it easier to give up punishment and get on with forgiveness—a great opportunity to hear the message in guilt and discover the power packed into love.

Look back through history. Which nations were quickest to mobilize and declare war? It's the same with individuals. You and I battle controlling behavior only when it highlights a personal fault that we've yet to forgive.

Often, we don't forgive ourselves for going into battle in the first place—because that choice always produces pain. (Can you and I forgive humankind for all their decisions to go to battle? General amnesty?) Breathe!

~ ~ ~

Experiment #87

The Forgiveness Mantra

This procedure, created out of Leonard Orr's Rebirthing therapy, is based on the exchange in Luke 18:21-22. Simon Peter: "If my brother sins against me, should I forgive him up to seven times?" Jesus: "Not seven times, but seventy times seven."

1. Construct an affirmation along these lines: "I (*your name*) now fully forgive (*myself or another*) for (*a specific offending action, thought or behavior*)."

2. Spend some time creating and rewording your affirmation until it resonates within you.

3. Once you feel that it's precise and completely accurate, write it out seventy times a day—for seven days. As you write, be aware of your feelings and emotions.

4. After the week is over, give thanks. What's changed in how you feel about the person or situation?

~ ~ ~

When mired in blame and revenge, ask the energy you've invested in those behaviors to nourish your ability to forgive. Whenever you're mired in self-contempt, ask the energy within that emotion to nourish your ability to love yourself. Ask the energy within your breath to nourish these ends as well.

~ ~ ~

Forgiveness includes both mental and emotional components, which is why it releases such incredible energy!

Whenever I need to forgive someone, there's always something in *me* that begs forgiveness. To start, I search for whatever pain I've hidden from myself. I need its message for my forgiveness to be complete—forgiveness always supports me in healing my pain!

Remember when my Volvo was rear-ended by that guy who wanted to berate me for my driving? It took me several days to forgive myself for having humiliated him in front of his family. That forgiveness required me to accept the experience as perfect—without having to justify my behavior. It taught me the sorrowful cost of punishing another person, even when I can justify doing so. It taught me that attacking anyone for *his or her* hostility doesn't work.

It taught me that I never need to blame others for making me feel diminished. (I can do that all by myself!) And . . .

It taught me the enormous value of supporting of others in pain, regardless of how I feel about them. And that one experience is helping me learn how to validate and love others without blaming myself for their pain, or taking on their blame.

Perhaps the first error you need to forgive is having diminished yourself. Consider that idea for seven days!

~ ~ ~

Forgiveness also requires that we trust—honestly! Unfortunately, we let ourselves be suspicious of each other—always with plenty of justifications, like *You haven't met my expectations.* In truth, your lessons have never been an impediment to my growing and contributing—quite the contrary. Perhaps trusting others starts with accepting them and their lessons.

Whenever I catch myself mistrusting someone, I find it empowering to meditate and ask my Higher Self, "What's needed to heal my distrust of *myself?*" Once I forgive my own shortcomings, suddenly I recover the ability to trust myself, and others!

So many times, I've pointed out to clients that their self-mistrust is reflected in their bodies. I ask them, "What would it take to trust your body to be a powerful healing ally?" And as we mistrust ourselves, so do we mistrust the universe. We mistrust pain and healing, we mistrust love. We mistrust the present moment. And the justifications we use are exactly the same ones we use to mistrust ourselves!

~ ~ ~

One of the most valuable lessons I've learned is that I can have fun with my challenges, rather than waiting until after the lesson is finished— this has immeasurably increased my trust of myself. Thus, I'm freer to trust people just as they are, without asking that they share—or behave according to—my standards. These days, if you and I have a problem, I'm more inclined to resolve it than to seek to invalidate you.

To forgive *effectively*, you must be willing to . . .

1) Trust that each and every one of us is divine, regardless of our lessons or behaviors.

2) Trust that pain is a valid healing event, and not a reason to blame anyone (including yourself!). Loving the facets of yourself you most dislike is one of the greatest challenges. But as you learn to do so (and thus heal these parts of yourself) you'll learn to appreciate others whom you've judged and condemned.

3) Trust that every event reveals the universe unfolding as it should, according to wisdom far beyond the grasp of our rational minds.

Journal Exploration #89

Trusting the Universe

1. Record a trauma or upsetting experience that still bothers you. Write down the circumstances of the event.

2. On a separate page, write down your emotional response to this event.

3. Were others involved in the event? Write down *their* emotional reactions, as best you recall.

4. Now imagine the same event, unfolding in a worst-case scenario. Briefly note the circumstances—and your emotional reactions.

5. Where in your body do these feelings occur? Breathe!

~ ~ ~

6. Listen for the message these feelings want to deliver.

7. What outcome would you like for this event? Define what you truly want. (Here's a good one: "I want to heal fear and my need to create similar events in the future.")

8. Connect with your feelings, and the energy within them. Ask them to support the manifestation of what you truly want.

9. Give thanks for the outcome—now, even though it's occurring at some future time.

10. Over the next several days, note any changes in your experience. Do you observe a greater awareness of your own capabilities? Give thanks.

11. Throughout the process, notice your constant opportunities to validate or invalidate yourself, regardless of circumstances. The universe delivers just the right experiences for us to grow and validate ourselves—and consequently, others.

Often unknowingly, we don't complete a lesson—we remain stuck in it. The energy of growth stagnates, and we miss out on the excitement of new challenges. And the best way to make sure you've completed a lesson is to give thanks for it.

~ ~ ~

Whenever you catch your mind suggesting a limiting or diminishing thought, replace it with an idea of gratitude. If you haven't great wealth to be thankful for, find something to appreciate—even if it's only the ability to balance your checkbook. I've found gratitude to be the most powerful of prayers—which most supports effective manifestation. I take great joy in giving thanks for my joys and pains, my lessons and the profound opportunities each of us has to contribute.

Perhaps loving ourselves and pursuing our ideals fervently is the greatest expression of gratitude to humankind (and God) possible.

~ ~ ~

The Hidden Energy in Blessing

During my marriage, I went through a period of conflict with my wife that seemed to persist for months. We fought, we cried, we prayed, we meditated, we talked, we withdrew, yet nothing seemed to be effective in moving through the conflict. This condition persisted so long that we jokingly referred to it as "Being stuck in Omaha."

One day in meditation, I finally got the bright idea of asking my Higher Self, "*Why* am I still stuck in Omaha?"

To which my Still, Quiet Voice replied simply, "Ned, you've forgotten to bless it."

I wanted to protest! After all, I'd been suffering for quite some time. Surely someone in this deep a swamp didn't have the power to bestow blessings—to make anything sacred. But as I thought about it, that was the only point of view I hadn't explored. I shared that with my wife and did offer a blessing of gratitude for the experience. And immediately the conflict lifted.

That helped teach me an important lesson: that I don't need to *like* a condition in order to bless it. As children of God, each of us has the power to bestow sanctity to any part of our lives. This lesson furthered trusting my Higher Self, so that often I ask the inner realms to support me in blessing some dimension of myself.

Experiment with blessing your dream self, whenever there's a painful event in that dimension!

Experiment #91

Find three different ways to give thanks and bless . . .

1. Yourself and the many dimensions of you.

2. Your own unique validity.

3. Your pains, joys, wants and desires.

4. Your unique contributions.

5. The most important current lesson in your life.

Repeat this exercise daily for twenty-one days.

We are each meant to be the sole and powerful guardian of our validity and sacredness. We are sacred stewards of our unique right to make choices—power that ultimately creates our reality. As we learn to let this life love us, we learn more of our power to bless and hold sacred the universe that holds us. So does the evolution of Heaven on Earth unfold.

~ ~ ~

Final Words
(for now)

Imagine a world where any two people could approach each other and immediately engage in a healing process. Where we all acknowledge the power to heal, and can explore pain with the intent of expanding our consciousness. Where we each seek this greater intimacy within our communities, expanding the joy of sharing our gifts, knowing the power that each of us has to hold ourselves inviolate. Where the human potential we're all impatient for, could finally manifest. What would our dreams for growth look like then?

Meanwhile ...

You and I are learning from each other.

We're learning to trust our own greatness—the unlimited God Within. We're learning to love the unknown self, thus nurturing the evolution of consciousness. As we pursue our ideals for humankind, we learn to serve the God Within Each Other.

We each sit on a gold mine of energy, awaiting our direction to manifest what we truly want.

We each have a unique gift to help bring about Heaven on Earth, yet we often use our power to create pain, lack and limitation.

Yet each painful lesson holds within it the energy to lead us back to Heaven on Earth.

May you take great joy in ...

Further discoveries of your own power,

The freedom of giving up control,

Letting your love and passion to contribute lead the way,

Trusting humankind to be a magnificent collaboration to present exactly those lessons you're needing for the unlimited expressions of God that are your potential,

Learning to trust your greatness,

Loving yourself as you explore this dance!

~ ~ ~

787 - 862 - 7771

508 - 457 - 1802

"Daved Godding"

Taylor Water st

)l hr

Vick 385 - 6227

11
10
110
5
550

2
550
22 00

550
250
800

16
3
29
8
23 2
464
464
928
2200
3,28